1997

Legal
the Integrated
Delivery System

An Executive Guide

American Academy of Healthcare
Attorneys of the American
Hospital Association
Deborah A. Randall, Esq., Editor

AHA
AHA books are published by American Hospital Publishing, Inc.,
an American Hospital Association company

This publication is designed to provide accurate and authoritative information in regard to the subject matter covered. The views expressed in this publication are strictly those of the authors and do not necessarily represent official positions of the American Hospital Association. If legal advice or other expert assistance is required, the services of a competent professional should be sought.

Library of Congress Cataloging-in-Publication Data

Legal issues and the integrated delivery system: an executive guide /
   American Academy of Healthcare Attorneys of the American Hospital
   Association ; Deborah A. Randall, editor.
       p.   cm.
   "A condensed version of . . . Hospital-affiliated integrated
delivery system"—Pref.
   Includes bibliographical references (p.   ).
   ISBN 1-55648-159-4
   1. Managed care plans (Medical care)—Law and legislation—United
States. 2. Medical care—Law and legislation—United States.
I. Randall, Deborah A. II. American Hospital Association. American
Academy of Healthcare Attorneys. III. Hospital-affiliated
integrated delivery system.
KF3825.L43 1996
344.73'03211—dc20
[347.3043211]   96-8090
                                         CIP

Catalog no. 118119

© 1996 by American Hospital Publishing, Inc.,
an American Hospital Association company

Printed in the USA

AHA is a service mark of the American Hospital Association used under license by American Hospital Publishing, Inc.

Text set in Sabon
3M—06/96—0437

Deborah A. Randall, Esq., Editor
Arent Fox Kintner Plotkin and Kahn

Audrey Kaufman, Senior Editor
Nancy Charpentier, Editor
Peggy DuMais, Production Coordinator
Marcia Bottoms, Books Division Director

Contents

Preface

Of the many trends that have fashioned new systems and forms of health care delivery, the trend to "integrate" the various delivery components across the continuum of care may have the greatest impact on the basic structure of the health care system in our country. The catalyst for integration is the increasingly rapid movement toward managed care and managed reimbursement methodologies. The traditional fee-for-services system of independent physicians, hospitals, and other providers is quickly becoming obsolete.

The seed of these changes was planted over 20 years ago with the implementation of Medicare's prospective payment system (PPS) in 1983. PPS created an incentive for hospitals to treat Medicare patients more efficiently and cost-effectively through the use of prevention programs, more effective treatment protocols, alternative and less expensive providers, and case management techniques. Soon other payers began to review the traditional fee-for-service payment system and moved to increase managed care requirements such as utilization review, preauthorization, and limitations on emergency room and other benefits provided by traditional indemnity insurance products. Now payers insist that hospitals and other providers accept per diem or capitated payments and thereby a greater portion of the financial risk of providing health care services.

To be able to efficiently address the managed care requirements, accept the increased financial risks, and maintain high quality care standards, hospitals are developing integrated delivery systems (IDSs) to coordinate the delivery of health care among hospitals, physicians, and other providers. This book is designed to assist nonattorneys at the highest levels of hospital management in their formation and operation of an IDS. Its purpose is to provide an overview of the key legal issues involved with a hospital-affiliated IDS.

In general, an IDS includes any organization or system of relationships among providers that involves the coordinated delivery of health care by its providers. It may or may not include hospitals in a governing or ownership role; however, by actively participating in the control and governance of IDSs, hospitals are in a better position to control their own destiny. Also, an IDS may or may not include a financing or insurance component. The degree of integration may be slight, as it is with most management service organizations (MSOs), or complete, as it is with a staff or group model health maintenance organization (HMO) such as Kaiser Permanente or Group Health Cooperative. The extent of integration depends largely on the demands of the marketplace and the willingness of providers to modify their traditional methods of providing services. Determining the form of that integration requires good faith, open negotiation by the participants, and resolution of the legal and operational issues discussed in this book.

Advice of legal counsel should be obtained in the formation of any new IDS entity, the funding of that entity, the division of ownership interests in the entity, development of the governance structure, and establishment of contractual relationships between the new entity and the participating providers. Hospitals will confront issues involving, among others, antitrust, tax exemption, pension and benefit, insurance and HMO licensure, fraud and abuse, self-referral, reimbursement and payment, the corporate practice of medicine, and security registration. This book discusses all of these issues as they relate to IDS formation and operation.

Acknowledgments

This book is a condensed version of an American Academy of Healthcare Attorneys' handbook entitled *Hospital-Affiliated Integrated Delivery Systems: Formation, Operation, and Contracts Handbook.* Two individuals need special recognition for helping transform the original handbook into this condensed version for health care executives and for supporting the editorial process: Jeffrey M. Sconyers, Children's Hospital and Medical Center, and Nancy J. Severson, Lutheran Medical Center. Both books are the result of the experience, insight, and hard work of the following task force members of the Academy's Managed Care and Integrated Delivery Systems Committee:

Douglas E. Albright
Ogden Murphy Wallace
Seattle, WA

Kathleen Sutherland Archuleta
Lutheran Medical Center
Wheat Ridge, CO

James M. Barclay
Cobb Cole and Bell
Tallahassee, FL

Thomas W. H. Barlow
Barlow and Lange, PC
Troy, MI

Clifford E. Barnes
Epstein Becker and Green, PC
Washington, DC

Jerry A. Bell
Fulbright and Jaworski
Houston, TX

Walter E. Bissex
Winstead Sechrest and Minick, PC
Austin, TX

David Bongiovanni
Cohen Shapiro Polisher Shiekman
   and Cohen
Philadelphia, PA

John D. Box
Duke, Branch, Box and Huber
San Antonio, TX

David S. Boyce
Jones, Day, Reavis and Pogue
Los Angeles, CA

Phyllis Brasher
Jenkins and Gilchrist
Dallas, TX

Bernadette M. Broccolo
Gardner, Carton and Douglas
Chicago, IL

Gregory A. Brodek
Kozak Gayer and Brodek
Bangor, ME

Laura L. Cross
Miller, Dollarhide, Dawson
   and Shaw
Oklahoma City, OK

Andrew J. Demetriou
Jones, Day, Reavis and Pogue
Los Angeles, CA

Eric E. Doster
Foster Swift
Lansing, MI

Diane Fisher
Hinkle, Cox, Eaton, Coffield
   and Hensley
Albuquerque, NM

Dennis J. Gallitano
Coffield Ungaretti and Harris
Chicago, IL

Peter N. Grant
Davis Wright Tremaine
San Francisco, CA

Peter H. Harris
Bryan Cave
St. Louis, MO

David C. Hillman
Verrill and Dana
Portland, ME

Robert Homchick
Davis Wright Tremaine
Seattle, WA

Daniel E. Hoodin
VHA Tri-State, Inc.
Indianapolis, IN

Gabriel L. Imperato
Broad and Cassel
Fort Lauderdale, FL

Michael C. Jones
Brown and Bain
Phoenix, AZ

Jeffrey P. King
Haynes and Boone, LLP
Dallas, TX

William A. Knowlton
Ropes and Gray
Boston, MA

Edward J. Krill
Carr Goodson and Lee, PC
Washington, DC

Melanie S. Lapidus
Sisters of Mercy
St. Louis, MO

Donna A. Lavoie
Barlow and Lange, PC
Troy, MI

Barbara H. Lebow
Saint Joseph's Health System
Atlanta, GA

Karin J. Lindgren
Sedgwick, Detert, Moran
   and Arnold
Chicago, IL

Gary J. McRay
Foster Swift Collins and Smith, PC
Lansing, MI

Patricia T. Meador
Bass Berry and Sims
Nashville, TN

Tecla A. Murphy
Coffield Ungaretti and Harris
Washington, DC

James Franklin Owens
McCutchen, Doyle, Brown
   and Enersen
Los Angeles, CA

Karen Carter Owens
Lewis and Roca
Phoenix, AZ

Ellen P. Pesch
Katten Muchin and Zavis
Chicago, IL

William A. Prince
South Carolina Hospital
   Association
West Columbia, SC

Kim H. Roeder
Powell, Goldstein, Frazer
   and Murphy
Atlanta, GA

Stanley W. Rosenkranz
Shear Newman Hahn
   and Rosenkranz
Tampa, FL

Douglas C. Ross
Davis Wright Tremaine
Seattle, WA

Chris Rossman
Honigman Miller Schwartz
   and Cohn
Detroit, MI

Anita F. Sarro
Bulkley Richardson and Gelinas
Springfield, MA

Donald R. Schmidt
Carlton, Fields, Ward, Emmanuel,
   Smith and Cutler, PA
Tampa, FL

Jeffrey B. Schwartz
Cohen Shapiro Polisher Shiekman
   and Cohen
Philadelphia, PA

Jeffrey M. Sconyers
Children's Hospital and Medical
   Center
Seattle, WA

Nancy J. Severson
Lutheran Medical Center
Wheat Ridge, CO

Stephen J. Sfekas
Weinberg and Green
Baltimore, MD

Thomas A. Sheehan, III
Moyle Flanigan Katz FitzGerald
   and Sheehan, PA
West Palm Beach, FL

David G. Sheffert
Coffield Ungaretti and Harris
Chicago, IL

Max Shelton
Harris Shelton Dunlap and Cobb
Memphis, TN

David S. Sokolow
Cohen Shapiro Polisher Shiekman
   and Cohen
Philadelphia, PA

Terence W. Thompson
Gallagher and Kennedy
Phoenix, AZ

John E. Steiner, Jr.
American Hospital Association
Chicago, IL

Donald P. Wilcox
Texas Medical Association
Austin, TX

Rhonda G. Teitelbaum
Rothgerber, Appel, Powers
   and Johnson
Denver, CO

Robin Wilson
Fulbright and Jaworski
Houston, TX

Martin J. Thompson
Riordan and McKinzie
Los Angeles, CA

Stephany S. Wilson
University of New Mexico Health
   Sciences and Services
Albuquerque, NM

These books reflect the hard work and expertise of these individuals in the numerous legal areas affected by the development and operation of integrated delivery systems. It also reflects their generosity in devoting the time and effort necessary to complete this lengthy project.

Chapter 1 ══════════════════════════════════════

Forming an Integrated Delivery System

═══

This chapter discusses the purchase of, or affiliation with, physician practices; the creation of new management service organizations (MSOs) and physician–hospital organizations (PHOs); and the special situations involving single-hospital and rural communities.

Hospital–Physician Integration

The key component in most integrated delivery systems (IDSs) is the integration of physician services.

Affiliation with Independent Physician Groups

Arrangements with independent physician groups that accomplish all of the hospital's and the physicians' objectives are difficult to structure, as the following discussion indicates.

Key Characteristics of Independent Physician Practices

Typically, independent physicians own all partnership interests or shares of stock in the professional partnership or corporation in which they practice medicine. Frequently, they also own, either individually or through their professional partnership or corporation, stock in an independent practice association (IPA) or an MSO in which they participate. A physician group may acquire practices by admitting partners to its partnership or issuing shares of stock in its professional corporation in exchange for the assets of any new physician joining the group.

A key business question for most physician groups is whether the physicians in the group will be willing and able to finance the growth of their group through individual guarantees of their portion of the group's debt.

The need for additional capital, and the limited ability of the group to finance this need independently, leads many groups to seek an outside capital partner. This need for capital creates an opportunity for the hospital to engage in partnership arrangements with the physician group. Often, however, physicians do not want to share ownership or control of their organization with the hospital. The hospital must then determine whether and how it should affiliate with the independent group—for example, as a lender or management entity, or by contracting with the group to perform certain services.

Key Characteristics of a Clinic without Walls/ Group Practice without Walls

This concept means different things to different people. Here, it is used to refer to a large, multilocation medical group. Physicians can exclusively own, control, govern, and fund the organization, or, in exchange for outside capital, may share ownership, control, and governance with the hospital. One of the key questions for physicians is whether they retain their existing practices, practice assets, employees, fee-setting authority, and autonomy over managed care contracts—that is, whether they actually merge their practices into one entity or remain organized as separate practices that share certain services or operate collectively as an IPA. Depending on state corporate laws, the legal structure might take one of several forms—professional association or corporation, limited liability company or partnership, or non-profit corporation or foundation.

The group practice without walls can be formed by a contribution of assets from existing practices. Either at start-up or later, the entity usually will need capital from another source. Therefore, the physician group will need to consider whether it needs a capital partner. A key consideration in assessing the group's capital needs is whether the group will be able to manage the risks of fixed, or capitated, payments from third-party payers. The hospital's dilemma is whether and how to affiliate with a group practice without walls.

Hospital Service Agreements with Independent Physician Groups

Traditionally, hospitals have contracted with independent physicians for hospital-based physician services or to serve as medical directors. Increasingly, however, hospitals are entering into various types of agreements with independent physician groups for coverage and operating arrangements. For example, a hospital might contract with a physician group to provide medical services at clinics and facilities or within departments owned and operated by the hospital. These arrangements usually arise as a result of one of three circumstances:

1. The hospital purchases the physician group practice and converts it into a hospital clinic.
2. The hospital establishes a new clinic and contracts with an independent physician group to provide coverage.
3. The hospital contracts with the physician group to become the operator of an existing hospital department, clinic, or facility.

Hospitals also might enter into agreements with independent physician groups for joint marketing and services. For example, the hospital and the physician group might agree to jointly seek managed care contracts. The hospital might enter into an agreement to provide administrative and management services to the physician group in exchange for a reasonable fee. The physician group also might designate the hospital as its marketing agent for managed care contracting purposes.

These service relationships are often referred to as MSO arrangements; however, some MSO arrangements provide further integration with the MSO (either owned solely by the hospital or in a joint venture with physicians) purchasing the tangible assets of physicians' practices, paying development costs, providing start-up and operating capital, and contracting with the group to provide office space, equipment, personnel, and management services. Sometimes independent physicians create a new organization to serve as an MSO for their practices.

Key concerns in the decision-making process for all of these service arrangements are financing and legal issues. The hospital needs to determine whether to pay for all of the developmental and organizational costs of the new marketing or practice management entity, or to share the costs with its physician partners. Furthermore, revenue-sharing and compensation arrangements for these service arrangements are particularly complicated and must be evaluated in light of Medicare anti-assignment provisions and state and federal laws prohibiting corporate practice of medicine, fee splitting, fraud and abuse, self-referral, and private inurement/benefit. In addition to these legal issues, these service arrangements must consider tax, licensure, managed care contracting, employment, insurance, antitrust, and other laws discussed in more detail in later chapters.

Another issue that is key to the success of these service arrangements is the allocation of power and authority between the hospital and the independent physician group. Key considerations are the duties and obligations of the parties to provide services to each other, the payment for those services, and the party that will employ, supervise, and pay for support staff. The hospital and physician group also need to decide whether the arrangement will be long-term or easily ended if it becomes burdensome or unworkable.

Finally, the hospital must determine whether the proposed contractual arrangements with an independent physician group will accomplish the hospital's goals and objectives with regard to critical issues such as physician recruitment, managed care partnership arrangements, and protection of its long-term interests, as well as whether they will possibly alienate other hospital medical staff members.

Hospital Loans to Independent Physician Groups

Hospitals might determine that it is advantageous to make loans to independent physician groups that participate with the hospital in operating clinics or providing other hospital services. The purposes of the loans might be for physician recruitment, equipment or leasehold improvements, working capital, or other purposes. If the loans are for physician recruitment, the hospital needs to determine whether a direct contractual arrangement should exist between the hospital and the recruited physician or whether the contractual arrangement should be solely with the physician group. Both the Internal Revenue Service (IRS) and the Department of Health and Human Services' Office of the Inspector General (OIG) are actively reviewing these arrangements. Federal and state laws and regulations governing fraud and abuse and self-referrals must be examined carefully to ensure that the arrangements are within available exceptions.

The hospital needs to consider whether it can legitimately achieve its purposes and protect its interests through restrictive covenants under the loans and whether this is the best mechanism for developing an affiliated practice entity. Key legal issues are similar to those involved in other contractual relationships between a hospital and independent physicians—for example, whether the loans provide a community benefit, whether they fall within available exemptions under the federal Stark laws governing self-referrals, and whether the terms of the loans are commercially reasonable. (The Stark prohibitions are discussed in detail in chapter 2.)

Joint Hospital–Physician Control of Group

The corporate practice of medicine laws of some states restrict stock ownership to persons who are licensed as physicians. To circumvent this restriction, a jointly owned and controlled hospital–physician entity might offer two classes of stock, one of which might be held by the hospital medical director (or other physician appointed by the hospital) and the other by other physician members of the group. The corporate documents could require that significant company actions have approval of the majority (or greater number) of both shareholder groups. Restrictions on transferring stock could affect both classes of stock. The hospital also might acquire control in the physician group's professional corporation or association by having the hospital medical director or other hospital-appointed physician hold the preferred stock, provided voting on significant issues is controlled by the preferred stock.

Key issues in evaluating these arrangements include state laws affecting the corporate practice of medicine and the structure and operation of professional associations and corporations, Medicare fraud and abuse statutes and regulations, the Stark laws, employee benefit and pension plan laws and regulations, laws and regulations affecting the hospital's tax-exempt status and capitalization of the corporate entity, federal and state antitrust statutes, and state statutes or case law affecting the enforceability of noncompetition covenants. Also, the tax consequences for the hospital medical director should be reviewed before he or she is asked to hold shares in the group on behalf of the hospital.

Hospital-Owned and Controlled Physician Group

Through ownership and control of a physician practice group, a hospital can attain a seamless continuum of care, develop databases necessary for effective utilization management, adopt risk-accepting price strategies such as capitation, and eliminate organizational barriers to more efficient delivery of care. In this structure, a hospital and a medical group are legally combined in a business organization as part of a single system. Either the organization may employ physicians directly or a separate entity may be established to deliver physician services to the organization. Typically, the organization will own the assets used by the practice and will manage the practice. The organization's success or failure depends on the governance and allocation of power among participants, the relationship between the hospital and the physicians both during and after the structure is developed, the mechanics of bringing the physician group into the employ of the hospital or hospital-owned entity, and the willingness and ability of all involved to work together cooperatively and effectively.

Opportunities

Historically, tension has existed between hospitals and medical staffs regarding resource allocation, fee structures, and other issues, even as there has been an incredible amount of cooperation in the delivery of patient care. Even though this tension can make hospital ownership of a medical group more difficult, market factors may provide incentives to both hospitals and physicians to facilitate hospital ownership and control of medical groups. A hospital-owned and controlled group will allow coordination of organizational goals and actions (including those relating to patient care) and establishment of financial incentives. A hospital-owned group may gain competitive advantages if other providers in the system's market are not able to offer a coordinated system. Economies of scale in management may arise from elimination of duplications in administrations and from the ability to offer "one-stop shopping." Better coordination of hospital and physician services, including communication of patient data, may lower the risk of malpractice with resultant lower insurance rates. Databases providing information on resource utilization belong to the system and allow it to lower, or at least more accurately assess, the risk of capitated price structures. Further, the integration attained by ownership will help address certain legal issues such as referral arrangements and antitrust.

Alternative Structures

Either the hospital or its corporate parent can employ the physicians directly, or a separate entity can be established as a medical services component for the integrated system. To a large extent, the choice of entity will depend on which entities are allowed to employ physicians under state law. In several states, the corporate practice of medicine prohibition precludes direct hospital employment of physicians or limits the choice of entity. (See chapter 2 for a discussion of the corporate practice of medicine doctrine.) Physicians may resist being employed directly by a hospital unless they are represented in the entity's governing body. To the extent that state law or physician attitudes prevent hospital ownership of the actual medical practice (as opposed to its operating assets), use of an entity to provide management and operational services is a common tool. Another alternative would be a hospital-owned clinic holding a long-term, exclusive staffing contract with a medical group.

Other factors that affect the choice of entity include limited liability, the nonprofit status of a parent company, capital-raising characteristics, and applicable tax law.

Alternative 1: Nominee Entity

Where direct hospital ownership of the entity used to employ physicians is not available due to state law or political issues, an indirect approach would be to acquire or create a traditional medical practice entity, such as a professional association or a professional corporation, with the support of an aligned physician. The physician should be dedicated to the hospital–physician integration concept, and generally be "allied" with the hospital (for example, hold a position such as medical director) or have contracted not to act independently of the hospital (for example, as a straw man or "nominee" to own the capital stock of the entity). The hospital could contractually bind the physician to vote and dispose of shares in the entity at the hospital's direction. However, care should be taken to avoid unintended adverse tax consequences to the allied physician shareholder.

Alternative 2: Nonprofit Corporation or Foundation

Certain state laws allow a nonprofit entity or foundation, of which a hospital is the sole "owner" or member, to engage in the practice of medicine.

Like any investor, the hospital typically reserves specific approval over certain decisions or actions, which might include:

- Operating and capital budgets
- Purchase and disposition of property
- Managed care contracting
- Loans
- Appointment of officers
- Incurrence of debt
- Addition and deletion of services or capacities
- Extraordinary transactions such as mergers
- Investment in other entities
- Election of directors
- Compensation

Key Consideration: Governance and Relationship with Physicians

To abide by state rules restricting the corporate practice of medicine, and to encourage the enthusiastic participation of physicians, the hospital could:

- Reserve executive officer position(s) for physicians
- Require a percentage of board members to be physicians, generally or by specialty
- Compensate physicians who accomplish integration goals, in addition to high levels of performance and quality performance
- Allow physician ownership of medical records

These physician rights raise important tax issues that are discussed in chapter 2.

Key Consideration: Method of Acquisition and Related Documentation

If permitted by state corporate practice laws, the hospital can buy the medical practice's capital stock or acquire its operating assets and employees. Alternatively, the hospital can start a new medical group that will acquire the practice's assets and employees.

In acquiring a practice and establishing relationships with the hospital-controlled medical group, the following documents will be among those needed:

- A stock or asset purchase agreement
- Articles, bylaws, and other organizational documents (if creating a new entity)
- Certification or licensure applications (if required by state law)

- An employment agreement for physicians (generally demanded by physicians but not necessary to establish an employment relationship)
- A buy–sell agreement and loan documents (if using a nominee entity)

Any purchase should be preceded by a "due diligence" investigation of the medical practice and its participating physicians.

The corporate documents should deal with possible issues of physician departures from the newly acquired medical group or the physicians' desire to repurchase the medical group. These include noncompete agreements (governed by state law), ownership and cost of delivering copies of medical records, and how (and whether) some or all of the assets acquired from the physician or his or her medical group may be repurchased if the parties terminate their relationship. If the new entity issues securities to make the acquisition, a shareholders agreement should address the possibility of unwinding the acquisition.

When the acquisitions involve an accumulation of market power, the acquisitions and recruitment together should be analyzed for antitrust concerns (discussed in chapter 2). The acquisition price and physician salaries offered by a tax-exempt hospital require consideration under the federal tax laws and fraud and abuse safe harbor regulations. State insurance and health maintenance organization (HMO) laws should be considered, and ownership and operation of the medical group must satisfy Medicare and Medicaid.

Foundation Concept

The medical foundation provides professional medical and related services directly to the public, usually as a hospital or a parent company affiliate. The foundation provides capital, equipment, office space, and management expertise, and often purchases the assets of individual providers and group practices. Depending on state law, the foundation either employs the physicians or independently contracts with a medical group to render service to the foundation's patients. Unlike an MSO, the foundation holds managed care contracts, bills and collects in its own name for services, and owns patient medical records and accounts receivable. The advantages are greater economic and operational integration and efficiencies among the providers, the foundation, and the related hospital(s). If federally tax-exempt under Internal Revenue Code Section 501(c)(3), the foundation avoids many federal, state, and local taxes, and may utilize tax-exempt financing.

However, the foundation model is a complex arrangement and physicians usually are concerned about loss of control over their practices. Even employed physicians cannot be required to refer only to providers within the affiliated system. Thus, system loyalty remains a critical element for success in the formation of a foundation model.

Corporate Characteristics

Subject to state law, the foundation may take any corporate form permitted to provide professional services. Some issues to consider include:

- To be tax-exempt, foundations must meet state and federal requirements, which limit (among other things) how much equity or membership the hospital can extend to others.
- Depending on state corporate practice of medicine laws, the foundation may need professional services agreements with providers who will deliver services to foundation patients.
- If possible, the foundation should be organized to avoid state licensure requirements.
- The foundation should control contract relationships with payers by obtaining its own provider numbers. (Payers may require a provider's board of directors to be controlled by a majority of direct service providers [that is, physicians], which may preclude tax exemption.)
- The Health Care Financing Administration (HCFA) allows payment only to an employer or to an organization in whose facilities the physician practices "exclusively."
- Obtaining a provider number as an "additional location" of the medical group destroys a foundation's independent provider status.
- Becoming the medical group's billing agent involves legal burdens and creates more of an MSO than an integrated provider organization.

The Tax-Exempt IDS Foundation Structure

Various IRS rulings suggest that certain factors are necessary for tax-exempt status. These include:

- *Accessible care:* Emergency rooms, urgent care services, and other services of a hospital are open to anyone regardless of ability to pay; services of a foundation must be available on the same basis to qualify for tax exemption.
- *Open medical staff:* The IDS hospital medical staff is open to all qualified applicants. (This position is changing because capitated IDSs need to control costs.)
- *Control:* The board of directors of the exempt organization is composed of no more than 20 percent physicians, and there are restrictions on physician committee representation (with the exception of committees dealing with medical affairs.)

    This limitation may run counter to some payer requirements for direct provider control to obtain a foundation provider number. One solution would be to have a majority of physicians on the board of directors but restrict certain powers, such as budgetary approvals and fee arrangements, to the nonphysician board members; however, the Internal Revenue Service may consider this an aggressive approach. Some state laws do not permit a board of a nonprofit corporation to have its majority be persons compensated by the company.

* *Noncompete agreements:* The IRS has questioned covenants not to compete from a community service perspective, but recognizes the business rationale for agreements that restrict provider ability to enter into contracts with parties that compete with the foundation.
* *Participation in Medicaire and Medicaid:* The foundation must participate in government programs in a nondiscriminatory manner, including acceptance of elective fee-for-service beneficiaries in foundation facilities.
* *Medical education, public education, and clinical research:* Key benefits the foundation can provide to the community are programs of public education, medical education, and clinical research.
* *Directed admissions:* Contracts between the foundation and medical groups should not include requirements to hospitalize patients in any specific facility unless pursuant to appropriate guidelines imposed by managed care contracts.
* *Charity care:* Certain annual levels of charity care are a significant requirement for tax exemption.
* *Acquisition of assets:* Whenever a foundation acquires assets from physicians, it must be done on an arm's-length, fair market value basis. It is important to note that payments for the purchase of *intangible* assets are closely reviewed and may be suspect under both private-inurement/private-benefit tax laws and the antifraud and abuse laws (even if technically permissible).

Fraud and Abuse, and Stark Legislation

Regardless of the form the foundation takes, concerns will be raised under Medicare and Medicaid fraud and abuse statutes, as well as under the self-referral prohibitions imposed by the Stark legislation which took effect on January 1, 1995 (Stark II).[1] Under the fraud and abuse statutes, transactions falling outside a safe harbor are not prohibited automatically, but the same is not true under Stark II. Any economic relationship that falls within the statutory prohibition and does not fit one of the express exceptions will absolutely prohibit a provider from referring patients in the manner the foundation expects. In the fall of 1995, Congress introduced with its budget reconciliation bill modifications to Stark II that would reduce the scope of Stark II.[2] These modifications have not been enacted as of publication.

Antitrust

Antitrust issues are raised by the interaction of the foundation with its related hospitals and other affiliates. Joint negotiations by the hospital/parent and the foundation with third-party payers may raise antitrust issues unless the foundation is considered a subsidiary or sister of the hospital/parent. Depending on foundation (and hospital) size and market share, certain practices should be avoided. Regardless of their form or relationship with hospitals, foundations would be well advised to adopt an antitrust compliance program when engaged in joint managed care negotiations. Chapter 2 contains more information on antitrust.

Pension and Employee Benefits Plans

If the foundation contracts with a medical group, there may be federal tax qualification issues for employee benefits plans of both the group and the hospital. See chapter 2 for more information.

Implications for Tax-Exempt Financing

When a foundation obtains provider services through an independent contractor relationship, its efforts to seek tax-exempt financing may be affected because the use of tax-exempt financed facilities by private individuals is restricted.

Management Service Organizations

An MSO provides managerial, administrative, and support services (which may include facilities and staff) to medical group practices of various types, including IPA group affiliations. MSOs are separate from the medical practices they serve, do not own the patient records, are not licensed providers of medical care, do not engage in medical practice or provide medical care directly to patients, may not be able to employ physicians (and perhaps other licensed providers), are not subject to JCAHO (Joint Commission on Accreditation of Healthcare Organizations) oversight, do not require a certificate of need, and, generally, are unregulated. However, these are general statements and the laws of the state jurisdiction should be reviewed carefully.

A number of hospitals or hospital systems have established medical group–related MSOs, and some have formed joint venture MSOs with their medical staffs. A few larger, entrepreneurial, freestanding (not directly associated with a hospital or health care system) MSOs have been able to gain access to the capital markets through public stock offerings (for example, PHYCOR).

In part, MSOs are back room or "service bureau" operations (billing, collection, and other management and administrative services), but in the IDS context, they can be much more. A comprehensive MSO might purchase some or all of the hard assets of the medical practices and provide the practice facilities, information systems, and personnel through a turnkey management service agreement (MSA). In this case, the medical practices remain the providers of medical care and retain the patient relationships, managed care contracts, and provider numbers; and the MSO (as agent) bills in the name of the medical practice. The MSO may be paid on the basis of a percentage of adjusted gross revenues, a cost-plus basis, a capitated basis, or a flat fee basis.

Structure of an MSO

MSOs may be created as operating divisions of a hospital or hospital system; may be set up as a joint venture between physicians and hospital, or some other partnership-type arrangement; or may be incorporated separately, as either subsidiaries of a hospital/hospital system or entirely freestanding entities. Generally, MSOs that principally provide management services to independent physician groups are not eligible for federal tax exemption.

MSOs that are divisions of a hospital/health care system might have divisional physician committees involved in the governance and control of MSO functions. These arrangements must be handled carefully so as not to affect the hospital's tax-exempt status. Furnishing seed money and operating expenses for the MSO either through a loan arrangement or as an investment in the MSO entity could result in private-benefit problems if money is loaned to the MSO (directly or through a guarantee) at less than prevailing interest rates, without the usual collateral or protections for loans, or without a reasonable expectation of realizing a return on the investment. The tax-exempt hospital cannot provide services to the MSO and the physicians cannot receive services at less than fair market value or fair market rental. If an MSO operation is the principal or substantial activity of the tax-exempt provider, the level of private benefit to the medical group could result in loss of tax exemption. If an MSO is used as a physician-recruiting vehicle, and if exempt organization funds are involved, the primary beneficiary should be the community and not the medical group.

MSO Operational Issues

MSOs present a number of complicated operating issues.

Management Services Agreement

The management services agreement (MSA) defines the relationship between an MSO and the medical groups it serves. The MSA obligates the MSO to provide the medical group with administrative services (billing, collection, accounting, utilization review, quality assurance, managed care contracting, and information systems) and, commonly, with facilities and personnel as well. Hospitals may prefer short-term MSAs to provide these needed services to medical groups as an interim step while both sides explore more integrated models.

Payment arrangements may include a percentage of adjusted gross revenues, a flat fee, a capitation payment, or a cost-plus reimbursement. Alternatively, the MSA may establish a joint budgeting process to determine the MSO's fee, with payments due after a minimum ("base") physician compensation and MSO payment shortfalls considered in subsequent annual budget negotiations. If MSA payments become an indefinite subsidy to the physicians, private benefit (applicable to tax-exempt hospitals) and fraud and abuse issues become serious concerns for all parties.

The MSO may require the medical group to adhere to certain performance standards, including hours of operation, coverage, staffing levels, number of patient encounters by specialty, and other economic criteria.

The MSA agreement may give the hospital or the medical group approval rights over MSO appointment of key personnel, managed care contracting decisions, expansion of facilities, large capital expenditures, and the like. Finally, many closely integrated MSOs restrict the MSO and the medical group in their dealings with third parties through exclusivity agreements and through requirements by the medical group that its physician members not compete with the MSO system. Both these agreements depend on state law and, where appropriate, antitrust law.

The MSA should include a mechanism for periodically renegotiating key terms (such as *payment*) and for ending the relationship for specified reasons. The MSA should clearly state when and how renegotiation occurs (time intervals, market events, unilateral request, and so on), how long renegotiation must continue before invoking external assistance, what interim compensation process will be in effect pending resolution, and whether a qualified arbitrator can make a binding determination based on criteria identified in the MSA.

In states with strict corporate practice of medicine bans or practice license restrictions, an MSO may *not* do the following: set requirements regarding referral of patients to specific hospitals; establish medical group fee or internal compensation arrangements; direct quality assurance (QA), utilization, and peer review; implement staffing ratios; or dominate managed care contracting decisions. Some states may challenge MSA compensation under "fee-split" laws, which can involve the criminal code.

Medicare Reimbursement Issues

Medicare policy provides that, generally, a medical group may bill the program for services performed by ancillary personnel only if those services are performed under the supervision of the physician who either employs the ancillary personnel or shares a common employer with the ancillary personnel. Because an MSO often employs the ancillary personnel, the MSO could lease ancillary personnel to the medical groups to meet the intent of the law; however, this solution is not specifically within HCFA's present policies.

The MSO cannot bill in its own name for the medical group's services. When acting as the group's billing agent, the MSO must not be compensated on a percentage basis and may need to be licensed under state law as a collection agency.

Antitrust Concerns

Under an MSO arrangement, the hospital and the medical group remain separate legal entities and may be considered competitors for outpatient care. Any managed care contracting within the MSO must comply with the antitrust laws relating to price-fixing, market division, refusals to deal, and monopolization. If an MSO becomes part of a true risk-sharing arrangement, the parties may be able to negotiate joint capitation rates or withhold arrangements with much lower antitrust risk.

Fraud and Abuse Concerns

Frequently, hospital-sponsored MSOs are structured to bring together and support primary care practitioners through beneficial management fee arrangements and wraparound recruitment and retention programs, both of which are under close review by the OIG. Below-market charges for MSO services raise the risk of fraud and abuse challenges under state and federal law (as well as private-benefit challenges under federal tax law).

MSOs that exist as wholly owned subsidiaries or divisions of a hospital are vulnerable to inadvertent Stark II violations when they enter into contractual relationships with medical groups whose members are referring physicians. Because this MSO structure would almost certainly involve Stark II "compensation arrangement," the physicians would violate the law when they saw patients at the hospital, which creates obvious problems.

The second Stark II issue that may arise in the MSO context relates to the provision of certain ancillary services by the medical group. To the extent that a medical group wants to continue to provide ancillary services under the in-house ancillary services exception to Stark II, it must continue to employ certain personnel who might otherwise be employed by the hospital through the MSO, thereby losing one advantage of centralized MSO services.

MSO Acquisition of Medical Group Assets

In most cases, the MSO will acquire all of the medical practice's tangible operational assets, such as inventory, equipment, and real property (including leasehold estates and improvements). However, the MSO will not be acquiring the entire medical practice. Because of the requirements of the Stark laws and applicable state antireferral prohibitions, the MSO should carefully consider (1) which, if any, assets relating to ancillary services will be purchased from the medical practice, and (2) whether those ancillary services will then be provided by the MSO back to the physicians with whom the MSO has a management agreement.

State law may prohibit acquisition of some assets, such as medical records, managed care contracts, covenants not to compete, and other contractual rights. Additionally, these assets are more likely to raise illegal remuneration issues.

Several valuation methodologies can be used in an MSO acquisition of a medical practice's assets. Accounting firms and consultants can be particularly helpful in the valuation process. Valuation is a subjective process and different approaches, used singly or in combination, may provide a range of values that can then be averaged or otherwise reconciled. Due consideration must be given in the valuation process to the antikickback, private-benefit and self-referral issues.

The *market appraisal approach* of valuing assets involves an analysis of historical purchases and sales of similar assets. This appraisal process may be difficult in valuing medical practices as a whole or as ongoing businesses, but useful for assets such as real estate, equipment, inventory, and so on. A *cost replacement valuation approach* uses the cost of reproducing or replacing the assets, but finding a medical practice's value based on its human assets may be hard (although not impossible) to value quantitatively. A *discounted future cash flow approach* uses a particular projected money flow, such as revenue, earnings, or cash, to calculate a present value of the cash flow to serve as an estimated value. Finally, a practice may be valued based on a *multiple of historical earnings*. However, because an MSO does not practice medicine, and thus cannot benefit from practice revenues, the money flow approach may not be an appropriate valuation methodology to use. Different methodologies can be used for different assets (for example, the market approach for real estate and furniture, and the money flow approach for leasehold interests and various contracts).

In purchasing any business, the buyer should investigate the assets thoroughly for completeness and accuracy of the seller's representations, legal barriers to the proposed acquisition (from shareholders, contract clauses, government regulations, and so forth), and liability issues such as environmental problems. If the MSO will be hiring employees from the medical practice, employee and benefit issues will have a greater significance. In all cases, the buyer should review medical malpractice claims, peer review actions, contracts of all kinds, stability of patient base, stability of employees, lease terms, collection experience, prior appraisals obtained by the seller, tax returns, and pension and other benefit plans.

If the purchaser or an affiliate receives referrals from members of the physician group or provides referrals to the practice group, any payment that is greater than fair market value raises issues under federal and state illegal remuneration laws and the nonprofit tax exemption standards. Independent appraisals and well-documented records of the fair market value paid for those assets minimize these concerns.

Under the Stark II law, a physician may not sell to a hospital-owned MSO (and MSOs owned by other entities engaged in businesses subject to the referral prohibitions) if the purchase and sale, or any continuing relationship that is part of the purchase and sale, constitutes a "financial relationship." Among the exceptions in the law are *compensation arrangements,* if the acquisition of a medical practice constitutes an "isolated transaction" at fair market value without taking into account, directly or indirectly, the volume or value of referrals between the parties. There is still an exposure if the MSO acquires assets for which it does not have any real need in the continuing business.

The agreement should provide for the seller's cooperation with the purchaser on various matters, including providing bills of sale for particular assets, assistance with accounts receivable (if purchased), notices to patients, and other appropriate actions facilitating transfer of the assets. Any arrangements for retaining current employees for specified time periods should be covered.

Other practical points to cover include:

- "Tail" insurance, purchased by the seller of the practice to cover claims arising out of incidents prior to the sale, unless the seller has occurrence coverage
- Repurchase agreements, should the MSO not meet the parties' expectations
- Procedures for the future treatment of patient records, including sensitive topics such as chemical dependency

Physician–Hospital Organizations and Managed Care Contracting Organizations

Many hospitals and their medical staffs are forming physician–hospital organizations (PHOs) to serve as a mechanism for the hospital and its physicians to contract jointly with HMOs, insurance companies, and self-funded employee benefit plans. The PHO also may perform peer review, QA, and utilization review (UR) activities on behalf of itself and selected payers. However, PHO participation does not necessarily preclude the physicians or the hospital from participating in ventures with other physicians or hospitals.

The PHO relationship emphasizes hospital–physician cooperation and cost-efficient medicine through:

- A unified entity to negotiate jointly contracts with third-party payers
- A structure for joint marketing
- UR and cost controls for which hospital and physicians are responsible to payers
- Incentives to control costs between hospital and physicians
- Increased operational efficiency of hospital and physicians to maximize revenues under third-party payer payment constraints

The PHO can undertake simple tasks such as negotiating the provision of particular services to specific payers on a fee-for-service basis or more complex functions such as organizing joint ventures to take advantage of investment opportunities. The basic model involves the PHO's negotiating contracts with third-party payers to provide physician and/or hospital services to the payers' subscribers. The PHO usually has authority (often through an administrator/broker) to enter into contracts that bind its members, which may range from straight fee-for-service (no risk assumption) to full capitation arrangements (substantial risk assumption). In some cases, physicians may be able to opt out of negotiated contracts. The PHO might permit the hospital, in affiliation with its physicians, to build a new facility or start a new service at an existing facility. The PHO might itself undertake such a venture, or it could plan and spin off a separate entity. Once contracts are in place, the PHO might service a UR or claims-processing function, if permitted by state law.

Structure and Tax Treatment

A PHO that will contract primarily with third-party payers should generally be a corporation (rather than a partnership) to limit liability, utilize simpler legal documents, streamline decision making, and, where desired, be nonprofit (possibly tax-exempt). Because contract revenues are paid to the hospital and participating physicians for services rendered, PHOs seldom produce profits, making their federal tax treatment less significant.

Liability

Because PHO activities potentially affect the delivery of patient care and the finances of their participants, PHOs should usually be organized to limit the liability of their members. Typically this goal is most easily accomplished with a corporation, though liability issues can be managed to some extent in a general partnership. Limited partnerships are possible; limited partners who take no part in management have only their partnership investment at risk. Newer forms of organization that include limitation of liability, such as the limited liability company (LLC) or limited liability partnership (LLP) may be available depending on state law.

Organizational Issues

Key organizational issues should be agreed on by the parties to a PHO, including capital contributions, voting, governance, transfers of interest, allocation of profits and losses, and termination. These issues are difficult to negotiate when a new relationship between a hospital and physicians is just starting.

Tax Consequences

It is important to consider taxation of the PHO entity if the PHO intends to generate or accumulate profits for future investment. It should be noted, however, that most PHOs pass contract revenues directly to the hospital and physicians as payment for services, essentially generating no net income. For these "no-profit" PHOs, income generally is offset by PHO operating expenses and tax status is immaterial.

A taxable PHO corporation pays tax on corporate income before distributing profits to the shareholders as dividends. A tax-exempt hospital shareholder would not pay taxes on the dividends, but the physician shareholders of the PHO would be taxed on dividends. This "double tax" reduces the benefits of a successful PHO.

A PHO partnership or LLC is not taxed on its income, but each taxable participant pays taxes on its share, whether or not the income is actually distributed. A tax-exempt hospital affiliate would pay no taxes if the PHO activity is related to the hospital's charitable or educational purpose.

If the PHO attempts to qualify for tax-exempt status, it will usually be organized as a nonstock, not-for-profit corporation. The hospital and representatives of the physician group would typically be members of the not-for-profit corporation and would fund the corporation's capital needs through payment of dues, fees, or other assessments. As members, the hospital and physician group would elect the board.

Rulings from the IRS have been variable, depending on the purpose and function of the physician component of the organization seeking tax exemption. Hospitals should seek an expert tax counsel with a health background to pursue such a ruling.

To maximize the chances of obtaining tax-exempt status for the PHO, the participants should (1) not limit physician participation to hospital staff physicians, (2) ensure that the hospital retains control over any decisions about the delivery of health care, and (3) to the extent possible, demonstrate that the PHO benefits the community by providing greater access to health care (particularly for medically underserved groups), improving the quality of care in the community, and either reducing costs or limiting cost increases that might otherwise occur.

If the PHO fails to qualify for Section 501(c)(3) status as a charitable organization, it may attempt to qualify as a social welfare organization under

Internal Revenue Code Section 501(c)(4). If the PHO is analogized to an IPA, the IRS is unlikely to consider the application favorably.

Securities Laws

The application of state and federal securities laws needs to be addressed if the PHO is formed as a for-profit corporation and if the hospital and the physician group each contributes capital in exchange for stock. A nonprofit corporation (taxable or tax-exempt) would avoid those burdens but might be subject to limited supervision by the state with respect to liquidation or disposition of substantial assets.

Because one goal of the PHO is to encourage membership by physicians, expensive stock purchases often can dissuade physician participation. Further, if the PHO is unlikely to develop any value, it might be misleading to position it as an investment; physician shareholders will expect to see their stock appreciate in value. Finally, there are significant Stark II implications for physician owners of for-profit PHOs.

Governance

Normally, governance of a PHO is shared fifty-fifty by hospital and physicians. In a PHO corporation, the directors generally would include equal numbers of hospital and physician representatives (though equal voting also can be distributed among unequal numbers of directors). In a PHO partnership, or LLC, the general partners/LLC members would be the entities representing the two groups. Either group would have veto power over the decisions of the PHO, and the PHO bylaws, partnership agreement, or LLC operating agreement should provide for quick decisions (for example, a time limit on board approval of certain kinds of proposals). If the PHO does not pursue a proposal, either group should be able to pursue it independently.

The physician members of the PHO can participate as individuals or through a separate entity, such as an IPA. If they do not form an IPA to participate in the PHO, the individual physician members can be given the right to elect their share of the PHO directors.

Right of First Refusal

Often the PHO is provided with a first-refusal provision under which the hospital and physician members agree to bring all managed care contracts and other "new ventures" to the PHO for consideration before they undertake them on their own outside the PHO. For business and antitrust reasons, this right of first refusal should be limited to a defined period (such as 90 days) so that if the managed care payer cannot, or is not willing to, negotiate with the PHO, it can negotiate individually with the physicians and hospital. The right of first refusal prevents undercutting the PHO's purpose.

To make a first-refusal provision more successful, the PHO should define *new ventures* in a manner mutually acceptable to both physicians and hospital. New ventures might be billing and administrative services, a computer network among the hospital and staff physicians, or malpractice support. To protect the physicians from financial exposure, PHO acceptance of a new venture might require a super majority or even unanimous approval of the physician directors. If the PHO votes not to undertake a new venture, the initiating member or members should be free to undertake the venture outside the PHO. The right of first refusal is the only right that members of the PHO will have with respect to ventures conceived by the PHO constituents; the members will have no other right to financial participation or indemnification in projects declined by the PHO.

A *closed* PHO (one that will not involve the entire medical staff) should be spun off as a separate entity so that the resources of noninvolved physicians are not utilized.

Effect on Hospital's Tax-Exempt Status

The hospital and the physician group should minimize the risk to the hospital's tax-exempt status by ensuring that participation in the PHO furthers the hospital's charitable purpose. First, the PHO arrangement should provide that each party's capital contributions to the PHO are commensurate with any membership interests they may have. Second, the hospital should receive full value for its patient care services. The hospital should not, for example, deeply discount its rates offered through the PHO unless physicians do so as well. Strict controls should be implemented to ensure that income that would otherwise be due the hospital is not diverted to the physicians. Planning in this regard should take into account not only actual payments to physicians, but also indirect benefits to the physicians by virtue of the hospital's participation. For example, if the overall payer package negotiated by the PHO is more favorable than the sum of what the participants might have negotiated individually, the physicians should not receive a disproportionate amount of such increase.

A third measure for protecting the tax-exempt status of the hospital is to have the PHO provide a new medical service or improve medical access to the community. The IRS will take a very dim view of any arrangement that serves primarily to increase compensation to physicians without providing a corresponding increase in medical services or care to the community. Fourth, the hospital should demonstrate, to the extent possible, that participation in the PHO will lead to reduced costs.

Finally, the hospital should receive fair market value for any items or services that it provides to the PHO, including those provided during the start-up phase and ongoing staff and support services. Any loans from the hospital should be documented with a promissory note that includes arm's-length terms, carries a market rate of interest, and is adequately secured. Subsidization of a PHO by a hospital participant also may be susceptible to challenge as a form of remuneration under the antikickback law because physicians benefit from its managed care contracts and other services. Additionally, the PHO may be a compensation relationship between the hospital and the physician participants within the meaning of the Stark II referral limitations.

Integration Opportunities in Rural and Sole-Hospital Communities

For many years, reimbursement methods did not change in rural communities. Sliding fee or discounted fee-for-service arrangements were used, and physician practices remained small and highly autonomous.

Although rural community providers have resisted forming IDSs, out-of-state HMOs and other MCOs may now be pressuring them to contract on a capitated basis. The most common response is some form of network or alliance. Rural providers have a much greater incentive, and need, to develop a strong network alliance than their urban counterparts. A rural provider's failure to become affiliated with the one or two viable networks in its community could result in its economic failure.

From a rural physician's perspective, the appeal of a PHO is that it allows some degree of patient management autonomy (while sacrificing management and billing autonomy). From the hospital's perspective, the venture more closely aligns the physicians in the area with the hospital (thereby enhancing its continued operation). Establishment of a separate PHO entity gives both physicians and hospital a feeling of participating in a unique and separate venture while isolating certain liabilities of the venture. The distinction between participation in the PHO and membership on the hospital medical staff remains, and different credentialing standards apply. Rural and small community hospital boards typically prefer a nonprofit PHO entity status.

Antitrust Concerns

Among rural providers, one key concern regarding IDS formation is in the area of antitrust (discussed in detail in chapter 2). The rural market typically is dominated by one or two hospitals and a limited number of physicians. Because of the high level of market concentration already present in rural communities, any effort to establish an IDS among existing providers raises significant market concentration issues. The positive competitive effects of networking may be more difficult to identify and the dangers of monopoly may be more severe. Network providers may not be able to require exclusive agreements that preclude participation in competing networks.

When an IDS is organized in a rural area, there often is significant pressure to allow most or all providers to participate in the system. However, if more providers are brought into the network than are necessary to achieve its legitimate economic and health care objectives, this overinclusiveness may be viewed as monopolistic. On the other hand, if too many providers are excluded and network membership is necessary for survival, the exclusions may be challenged as a "group boycott." These issues can be addressed by making networks nonexclusive, allowing providers to compete outside the network and to participate in other networks. The provider network also should establish objective criteria for membership that relate directly to quality of care or achievement of economic efficiencies and that prevent competing providers from making specific membership decisions about each other.

Because an effective IDS in a rural area involves significant collaboration as to price and other market-related issues, the network must achieve a high degree of economic integration through the sharing of capital, risk, and reward. A "network" of providers without any shared risk is likely to be challenged under state or federal antitrust laws, unless providers effectively are removed from price and other competitively sensitive decisions. This removal, however, will weaken the effectiveness of the PHO.

Several states have enacted legislation expressly designed to facilitate cooperative arrangements among providers, particularly in rural areas. These state laws generally require prior review and approval of cooperative arrangements by the state governmental agency doing antitrust enforcement. However, ongoing supervision of the cooperative activity by the state agency varies, and it is unclear whether most states do enough active supervision to remove the providers' activity from review under federal antitrust laws. Therefore, participants should understand that state approval does not necessarily imply federal antitrust compliance.

Fraud and Abuse Considerations

In the area of fraud and abuse, the rural provider safe harbor requires the entity to offer the opportunity for investment in a good-faith, nondiscriminatory manner to any individual or entity that is a potential source of capital. However, this safe harbor may not work well for IDSs. Similarly, the additional safe harbor requirement that the entity must generate a high percentage of its dollar volume from servicing individuals who reside in the "rural area" may be so restrictive in its application as to nullify the benefits of the proposed safe harbor. Rural providers welcomed Stark II's exception that ownership arrangements related to entities in rural areas are not subject to the Stark II absolute referral prohibition if substantially all of the designated health services provided by the entity (including where a hospital and physicians are owners) are furnished to individuals who reside in a rural area.

Regulations published in 1995 applying to the clinical laboratory field suggest that an entity may be physically located in a nonrural area but furnish substantially all of its designated health services to individuals residing in a rural area and still qualify for the safe harbor.[3]

Reimbursement Incentives

Rural providers enjoy certain reimbursement incentives that are not available to urban providers. For example, providers in underserved areas can form either a rural health clinic (RHC) or a federally qualified health center (FQHC). A PHO could be eligible under these programs to receive a form of cost-based reimbursement if the geographic area in question is underserved.

The shortage designation regulations do not require designating the area using town or county lines; the designation need only have a rational basis. An RHC can be established for either a medically underserved area (MUA), a medically underserved population (MUP), or a health professional shortage area. However, only designation as an MUA or MUP will support establishment of an FQHC. One alternative for institutional providers is to carve out their emergency room and place it in the RHC or FQHC.

The Process of Physician Practice Acquisition

Physician practice acquisitions present several challenges and require substantial negotiation. Typical steps for the hospital buyer include the following:

1. Identify the acquisition opportunity
2. Conduct preliminary discussions
3. Form the acquiring company
4. Develop a deal structure
5. Execute a confidentiality agreement and a letter of intent
6. Perform a comprehensive due diligence review
7. Negotiate and execute a definitive acquisition agreement
8. Close, transfer assets and operations, and commerce new activity

These steps should be undertaken with an agreed-on timetable for the parties and with decisions made about which party (and counsel) will initially draft the acquisition agreement and other documents. Generally, control of document drafting can provide significant strategic and psychological advantages.

The Initial Build-or-Buy Decision

Initially, the hospital should decide whether to build or buy the physician practice necessary to create its desired vertical integration. That decision should consider the hospital's integration goals and strategy, and the internal and external environments. The internal environment includes the medical staff development plan, the hospital's strategic plan, an internal financial analysis linking existing hospital operations to projected integration system operations, and discussions with the affected physicians. The external environment includes the market plan; any analysis of competing hospitals, clinics, or physician groups; and any analysis of the managed care activities in the service area. A business plan will harmonize the hospital's previous analysis with the project and memorialize the factors and assumptions for entering the new business initiative of providing physician services. Weighing these considerations will better enable a hospital to determine whether it will be more effective to build physician practices from the ground up, to acquire practices, or to pursue a combination of build and buy to establish the base for an integrated system.

If the decision is to acquire physician practices, the existing analysis and/or business plan provides legal counsel with an important resource from which to outline the acquisition process, prepare the definitive acquisition documents, and review any inconsistencies with hospital decision makers. Counsel then will review and address the antikickback, self-referral, corporate practice of medicine, antitrust, tax, licensure, reimbursement, and Employment Retirement Income Security Act (ERISA) (including pension and personnel) issues in the transaction.

Physician Objectives

The physician seller's objectives may be harder for a hospital to determine, but understanding them is critical to structuring and negotiating a suitable deal. For example, whether the seller desires a taxable or nontaxable deal is one factor in determining whether to acquire the physician practice's stock or assets. If the seller is not opposed to an earn-out or deferred payment, applicable certificate-of-need obligations (if any) might be avoided. The hospital or IDS needs to know whether the seller's motivation is relief from regulatory, administrative, or capital concerns; access to management systems; new patient or revenue streams; or improvement of negotiating leverage with managed care payers.

Acquiring Entity

One of the initial determinations is whether the practice will be acquired by the hospital itself or by a separate entity. If the practice is a freestanding physician clinic, Medicare Part B reimburses physician services (and services and supplies furnished "incident to" physician services) under the Medicare physician fee schedule with no separate overhead reimbursement. Payment for physician services provided in a hospital-based clinic was lowered in the past by a site-of-service differential because the hospital was reimbursed on a cost basis under Medicare Part A for facilities charges at the clinic. As more outpatient services move under a Medicare DRG (diagnosis-related group), this situation will change; however, the differential in reimbursement must be factored into the acquisition decisions. The parties should seek expert advice to determine whether hospital-based clinic or free-standing clinic reimbursement will, in any particular situation, be more advantageous.

HCFA's regional office decides whether a clinic is hospital based or freestanding based on three threshold factors: (1) whether the clinic and hospital are licensed as a single health entity; (2) whether the clinic and hospital are subject to the bylaws and operating decisions of the same governing body; and (3) whether the clinic and its medical personnel are considered by the governing body to be subject to the rules of the hospital's medical staff. If these factors are unclear, information regarding common ownership and operational integration will be reviewed. Whether freestanding or outpatient, the hospital's interests are in maximizing reimbursement in keeping with other strategic goals.

If state law allows a non-physician-controlled entity to own a professional corporation (PC), the acquiring entity may be a PC owned in whole or in part by the hospital. If the buyer is restricted from owning the PC due to a corporate practice of medicine doctrine, one option is a PC in which the stock is held solely by a friendly physician who is controlled by the hospital buyer. A *friendly physician* can be any physician who is closely affiliated with and loyal to the buyer, not affiliated with the seller, and not subject to divided interests. Typically, this is a hospital employee or director, such as the vice-president of medical affairs or the medical director.

To exercise control over the friendly physician-shareholder, the hospital may want a stock transfer agreement that grants the hospital sole authority to designate another physician-shareholder should the first physician-shareholder cease to be employed, be affiliated, practice medicine, and so on. The agreement also could contain voting restrictions to ensure that the physician-shareholder votes his or her shares in a manner that is consistent with the interests of the buyer. Other restrictions could be placed in the PC's articles of incorporation and bylaws to require, among other things, super-majority votes for certain actions by the board of directors, and distribution rights in favor of the buyer in the case of liquidation of the PC.

If the IRS treats the buyer as the real owner of the stock of the acquired practice and the friendly physician-shareholder as a mere nominee or agent, significant consequences would follow and the organization's method of accounting would change from cash to an accrual basis. To avoid such adverse tax consequences, the buyer should allow the physician-shareholder to have governing control over the PC and to elect other physicians to the PC's board of directors. Further, the buyer could maintain control over only a minority of the board and intervene only in the most critical matters. Ultimately, however, the buyer should weigh the detriments of adverse tax consequences to loss of control.

Other Issues

Other issues for the nonprofit buyer include not funding a for-profit to a degree that would be considered a private benefit to the sellers. Arm's-length terms and fair market value pricing are essential.

Pension issues include the worst-case possibility that the hospital buyer and the PC will be considered to be under "common control," and thus the employees of both entities considered together to determine whether the pension or other benefit plans of the buyer and PC are unduly favorable to highly compensated individuals. See chapter 2 for more information on this very complex subject.

Structuring the Acquisition

There are three transaction forms for a hospital to acquire a medical practice: asset acquisition, stock acquisition, and merger or consolidation.

Asset Acquisition

In an *asset acquisition,* the hospital purchases all (or substantially all) of the seller's assets and, possibly, certain liabilities. Asset acquisitions also are utilized to acquire certain nonclinical assets for an MSO or a foundation.

The main advantage to an asset transaction is that parties can specify which assets will be acquired and which liabilities assumed. Buyers should be particularly aware of avoiding the inadvertent assumption of liabilities. To ensure that an asset transaction does not include liabilities for malpractice, the asset purchase agreement should provide that no liabilities other than those expressly identified are assumed. Other advantages include not needing to negotiate with individual shareholders and the assignment of a new tax basis by allocating a particular portion of the purchase price to a particular asset.

The main disadvantage to a seller is that gain from the sale of assets will be taxed to the seller at the corporate level and the proceeds will be taxed again upon distribution to the individual shareholders (assuming the seller operates as a corporation). It may, however, be possible to channel additional funds directly to physicians through such things as consulting agreements and signing bonuses (subject to fraud and abuse rules). Another disadvantage to an asset acquisition is that the transaction documentation is more complex because all assets to be transferred and liabilities to be assumed must be identified. Both buyer and seller must obtain necessary consents to transfer contracts to the acquiring entity, prepare documents to transfer leasehold interests or title to real property, and pay state or local transfer taxes.

Stock Acquisition

A *stock acquisition* is the purchase of all or a majority of the outstanding shares from the shareholders of a corporate seller. It avoids the double tax treatment of an asset acquisition. Some individual shareholders' stock receives long-term capital gain tax treatment. No transfers of specific assets or liabilities are required; they continue to be held in the name of the practice. The key drawback of a stock acquisition is the simultaneous acquisition of all corporate liabilities known and unknown. Although the liabilities remain in an entity that is separate from the acquiring entity, unfavorable contracts, litigation claims, and other business problems indirectly (and sometimes directly, as in environmental pollution claims) become problems of the acquiring entity. In addition, some contracts with payers, other providers, or others (such as banks) still may provide for approval or notice rights if there is a change of control. To give the buyer some protection, extensive due diligence should be conducted and individual shareholders of the selling entity should provide representations, warranties, and indemnifications as to outstanding liabilities. Indemnifications should be secured due to the difficulty of collecting, especially from shareholders who become employees of the buyer.

Merger or Consolidation

The third form of acquisition is merger or consolidation. A *merger* combines one corporation into another corporation with the surviving corporation assuming all of the property, assets, liabilities, problems, and obligations of the merged corporation. In a *consolidation,* two or more corporations combine to form a new corporate entity. A merger or consolidation avoids the necessity of numerous transfers of various assets and liabilities; it reduces the problems of minority shareholders. Some mergers can be structured as a tax-free reorganization, with no recognition of gain or loss at either the corporate or shareholder level.

Merger disadvantages include the assumption of all of the merged company's liabilities, obligations, and business problems along with its assets. As in a stock acquisition, the buyer should conduct extensive due diligence, and insist on extensive representations and warranties from the seller in the merger agreement. The buyer should also require that some or all of the seller's shareholders be liable personally for the seller's representations and warranties through an adequately secured indemnification mechanism.

Confidentiality

A confidentiality agreement should be executed prior to the initial due diligence investigation. This document balances the seller's need to protect its confidential or proprietary information and the buyer's need to acquire as much information as possible. When sales do not go forward, this agreement tightly restricts disclosure and use of the exchanged information.

In physician practice acquisitions, the protection of proprietary and confidential information is critical for both buyer and seller. When the practice group has other suitors or has significant market share, it may request information on the buyer's financial status, outpatient activities, and strategic plans. Sometimes the request is merely for "show"; other times, however, the seller actually wants to assess the hospital's view of the future, especially if the seller's physicians will continue to practice medicine with that buyer after the sale. The provider of information may want to delay the disclosure of the most sensitive information until after binding commitments have been made. When buyer and seller are actual or potential competitors, the parties may want to exchange current price or market information only after they have executed binding definitive commitments, and may want to use a third party to collect, analyze, and "sanitize" such information before disclosure in order to reduce antitrust risks.

Confidentiality agreements generally:

- Are limited to truly confidential information
- Limit access to specified personnel with need to know
- Restrict use of the information
- Provide for return or certified destruction of all exchanged documents and copies
- Provide a disclaimer that the information proffered may not be complete or otherwise reliable
- Provide that the recipient of information is responsible for the breach of the confidentiality agreement by any employee or agent
- Provide for an injunction to enforce it
- Provide that the agreement survives any termination of the acquisition discussions

Letter of Intent

Before entering into definitive agreements, the parties may enter into a letter of intent, also referred to as an *agreement in principle* or *memorandum of understanding*. This states the essential terms agreed on, identifies the outstanding issues, creates an ethical commitment of the parties, and may ease the negotiations toward a final agreement. It may contain binding obligations relating to publicity, allocation of expenses, limitations on negotiations by the prospective seller with other potential buyers, and limitations on major actions a party can take that would affect its status adversely. A letter of intent generally states the parties' intentions to avoid any fraud or tax issues.

A letter of intent also usually limits or totally restricts any public announcement until after the deal is substantially completed. Generally, letters of intent state they are not binding (enforceable). If buyer and seller intend to have a completely or partially binding letter of intent, a clear statement specifying the extent to which the letter of intent is binding should be included. In either event, clarity is key.

In addition, the letter of intent should contain the business terms of the transaction, including the purchase price or formula, the payment structure, and the relative responsibilities for expenses for the deal. It also should describe the form of the transaction (stock or asset acquisition, or merger). Other provisions often included are: government or corporate approvals to be sought; due diligence procedures and time line; what adverse changes in business between signing and closing could allow termination; special arrangements with directors, officers, or employees; any binding provisions such as confidentiality, expenses, or publicity; and the timetable for completing the transaction.

Due Diligence

Initial due diligence prior to development of the projected deal structure assists the buyer in deciding whether to proceed with the transaction. The second part of due diligence occurs after the letter of intent is executed, but before the acquisition agreement is completely finalized. This review provides the buyer with sufficient information to understand the business it is acquiring and the obligations it is assuming. Stock acquisitions and mergers require far more comprehensive due diligence evaluation than asset acquisitions.

For medical practices, due diligence typically evaluates, among other areas:

- Litigation
- Insurance policy coverage continuation
- Pension plan employer contributions
- Contract provisions on assignment or change in control
- Real estate and leases
- Compliance with applicable laws and regulations
- Liens and other encumbrances on practice assets
- Licensure, certification, and similar practice issues

Counsel will review many other documentary matters and may prepare an executive summary of significant issues that should be brought to the attention of management.

Definitive Agreement

The definitive agreement memorializes the agreement of the parties and typically will exist long after the signatories to the agreement have moved on. It should recite why the parties want to do the deal and how the transaction fulfills the community benefit or other purposes. It should be conceived as not just an agreement between the parties but also as an exhibit in a federal tax audit or fraud and abuse investigation.

Most medical practice acquisition agreements:

- Identify the parties, the assets, or the stock subject to the transfer; the consideration to be paid or the formula for determining the purchase price; and the closing timetable and mechanics
- Set forth the "representations and warranties" of the seller, the seller's shareholders, and, if appropriate, the buyer
- Describe the preclosing actions that each party agrees to do, or refrain from doing, between the execution of the agreement and the closing
- Set forth conditions that must occur prior to each party's being required to close the transaction
- Describe other provisions regarding indemnification, noncompetition, confidentiality, and medical records
- Describe the closing and termination of the transaction

The representations and warranties in an acquisition can be the hardest part to negotiate, and typically include statements concerning (as appropriate to the transaction):

- Organization, qualification, and standing
- No breach of enabling documents and contracts
- Corporate authorization
- Properties and leasehold interests
- Current ownership and stock rights
- Financial statements/taxes
- Events subsequent to date of audited statements
- Guaranties and contingent liabilities
- Professional licensure, certification, and medical staff standing
- Malpractice history
- Antikickback and self-referral compliance
- Litigation, investigations, legal compliance
- Employees/labor relations/ERISA
- Insurance
- Contracts
- Hazardous or toxic substances
- Corporate and government approvals
- Securities registration/exemptions

Buyer's counsel typically will want the representations and warranties to be broad and comprehensive and to survive the closing. Seller's counsel may want to limit representations and establish a time limit for claims under the agreement. Buyer's counsel may want to include indemnification provisions and other remedies in the event that the seller breaks promises in the definitive agreement and causes damages. Seller's counsel will want to build in a cap for such financial provisions.

The definitive agreement also should address medical record ownership, retention, and transfer, where necessary. Some states regulate medical record ownership and retention, and when the physician is an employee of a corporation, ownership of the medical record may lie with the employer corporation.

When the acquisition involves transferring the acquired practice to another physician, the American Medical Association (AMA) and some state medical societies require notification to active patients of the physician whose practice is being transferred, and that the physician with custody of the medical records send the records or copies to any physician designated by the patient, upon receipt of a written request. In such cases, the acquisition documents should include a sample letter of the announcement and a form authorization for the transfer of the records to another physician. A joint announcement sent to the seller's patients from buyer and seller together could implicitly promote the buyer. The goal, of course, is to keep the patients.

The definitive agreement should address whether the buyer wants any relocating physician to remain for a transition period to provide a personal introduction of the buyer (or the buyer's physician[s]) to patients. Part of the purchase price could be held in escrow and paid out over a transition period if doing so does not have adverse fraud and abuse consequences. Alternatively, the agreement could provide payment for consulting services provided by the departing physician during the transition period.

The definitive agreement also may include noncompete restrictions to protect the value of the medical practice acquisition. In some states, such covenants are valid only in connection with the sale of a business. Noncompete restrictions should:

- Be reasonable in duration
- Be reasonable in describing geographic areas that would affect the target's practice adversely
- Be reasonable in subject matter (only specialties in the target's practice)
- Include nonsolicitation clauses that do not limit a patient's right to freedom of choice
- Provide for enforcement provisions, including injunctive relief and liquidated damages

The Closing

Buyer and seller must determine whether to "close" at the execution of the definitive agreement or to schedule the closing after execution. When the closing is deferred, preclosing covenants will specify the conditions that must be satisfied before the transaction is consummated.

At closing, the parties deliver the documents conveying the physician practice, pay the purchase price (or deliver loan or other documents providing for delayed payment), turn over keys or similarly transfer possession, and pay closing settlement amounts. The parties may deliver other documents such as a corporate secretary certificate and certificates of good standing, articles, and bylaws. If the closing has been deferred, the parties also may deliver updates. Finally, to ensure that the transaction and the acquisition documents are legally enforceable, the parties may require legal opinions from each party's respective counsel. Legal opinions add to the cost of the transaction and may or may not provide significant additional protection.

References

1. *See* OBRA 1993 (42 U.S.C. § 1395nn), commonly referred to as Stark II.

2. *See* H.R. 2491, 103rd Congress, 2d. Sess. (1995).

3. *See* 60 Fed. Reg. 41914 (Aug. 14, 1995).

Chapter 2 ▭

Understanding the Legal Issues Affecting IDS Formation and Operation

▭

When hospital executives consider organizing or joining an integrated delivery system (IDS), they will quickly find that numerous legal issues must be addressed.

Antitrust Issues

Antitrust issues permeate any combination of providers in an IDS. This section reviews the statutory framework and important operational considerations in this area.

Statutory Framework

The antitrust laws grew out of "trust-busting" activities in the late 19th and early 20th centuries and are now embodied in a series of federal and state statutes.

The Sherman Act, Section 1

The Sherman Act, Section 1,[1] prohibits every "contract, combination . . . or conspiracy" that is "in restraint" of trade. As a general rule, a hospital and its officers, employees, and trustees are not independent from one another and cannot conspire for antitrust purposes. The same is true of a corporation and its wholly owned subsidiaries: They are considered one entity. Similarly, an integrated physician group practice is considered one entity and its members are considered to be legally incapable of conspiring with one another.

A violation of Section 1 requires an agreement that is unreasonably anticompetitive. Certain agreements are presumed in the law to be unreasonable (per se offenses) and a person's motives and intent, and the actual effect of the agreement, are irrelevant. Per se offenses include price-fixing, market allocation, and, in certain cases, group boycotts.

On the other hand, a practice may not constitute a per se offense, but still violate the Sherman Act under the "rule of reason," if it causes adverse economic results, such as an increase in price or a restriction in output. Defendants in these cases must show that the purpose *and* effect of the restraint are not to harm competition but that, on balance, the restraint is neutral or procompetitive.

The Sherman Act, Section 2

The Sherman Act, Section 2,[2] prohibits monopolization and attempts or conspiracies to monopolize. "Monopolization" means intentional acquisition of monopoly power, which is the power to control prices or production. Possession of monopoly power alone, if obtained or maintained by historical accident or business skills, does not violate the antitrust laws. Market definitions and control, conduct, and intent are important factors in these charges.

The Robinson-Patman Act

The Robinson-Patman Act[3] prohibits price discrimination in the sale of tangible goods, such as pharmaceutical products, when this activity substantially lessens competition or tends to create a monopoly.

The Clayton Act, Section 7, and Premerger Notification

The Clayton Act, Section 7,[4] prohibits mergers and acquisitions where the effect "may be substantially to lessen competition" or to tend to create a monopoly. Parties to certain mergers and acquisitions must notify the federal government in advance if the parties and transaction are of a sufficiently large size, as defined by the Hart-Scott-Rodino Act and its regulations.[5]

The Federal Trade Commission Act, Section 5

The Federal Trade Commission Act, Section 5,[6] enforceable by the Federal Trade Commission (FTC), makes unlawful "unfair methods of competition," which overlaps certain prohibitions in the Sherman and Clayton Acts. As a result, the FTC can take action to enforce these acts as well as its own act.

State Antitrust Laws

All states have antitrust laws that, to a greater or lesser degree, duplicate portions of the federal antitrust laws. Some state antitrust provisions go beyond the requirements of federal law.

Enforcement of Antitrust Laws on IDSs

IDSs are composed of a variety of health care providers, many of whom may be actual or potential competitors. The IDS may be organized as a single corporate entity such as a health maintenance organization (HMO). Alternatively, it may be structured as a series of corporations, partnerships, or some contractual form of provider network. The structure of the IDS and the degree of integration among its various components are critical elements in determining how the IDS is viewed under the antitrust laws. Whether an IDS will be viewed as one actor or several will determine the degree to which it will be able to contract collectively for its participating providers without running afoul of the antitrust prohibitions on price-fixing, market allocation, or group boycotts.

Several years ago, in the Supreme Court case, *Arizona v. Maricopa County Medical Society,* physicians lost their argument that medical society organizations that set maximum physician fees in insurance plans were legal under the antitrust laws.[7] Because the medical society physicians were not members of a true economic joint venture and because the physicians controlled a substantial market share, their price setting was illegal. To be a joint venture, the court said, providers must pool their capital and share risk to create a new, economically integrated entity. Courts will permit competitors to come together in a venture to provide a new or existing product in a more efficient manner, and will allow some secondary restraints if they are no broader than necessary to accomplish the venture's purpose.

The 1993 Statement of Antitrust Enforcement Policy in the Health Care Area[8] (the Antitrust Guidelines) promulgated by the FTC and the Department of Justice (DOJ) establishes guidelines for multiprovider networks, identifying a roster of positive features that might offset the negative aspects of collaboration. Networks that use capitation and payment withholds to achieve efficiencies are provided FTC/DOJ support.

Joint ventures among physician groups also are addressed by the Antitrust Guidelines. The "safety zone" established in this area applies to exclusive physician networks that are composed of 20 percent or less of the physicians, and to nonexclusive networks of 30 percent or less in each specialty practice, in the relevant geographic market. There have been numerous positive rulings from the FTC concerning very extensive physician networks; a few recent rulings have disapproved models with high market share, where the contract broker or messenger participates in the negotiations rather than simply conveying information between insurer/payer and individual physician/group.

The level of integration necessary for a multiprovider joint venture to be considered "safe" did not get a specific description in the Antitrust Guidelines. For physician networks, the federal agencies look for the presence of significant financial risk sharing to achieve cost containment goals, such as capitation or substantial withhold of compensation due to members. The same kinds of financial risk indicators were endorsed by the FTC and DOJ for multiprovider networks.

The enforcement agencies have made clear that much activity does not fall within the safety zones but may not be subject to challenge. Therefore, an IDS can be formed outside the safety zones but must take care when pricing IDS member services. Networks controlled by providers can easily be characterized as price-fixing agreements unless they take pains to integrate sufficiently and prove that the "efficiencies" of integration outweigh any anticompetitive effects of integration. Positive factors of integration include:

- Net efficiencies derived from operation of the network and passed on to consumers
- Assumption of financial risk
- Reduced administrative costs
- Improved utilization review
- Improved case management
- Quality assurance
- Economies of scale

IDS Managed Care Pricing

An IDS may contract with payers by several "mechanisms." From an antitrust perspective, the key is the extent to which the integrated providers share financial risk and promote cost containment.

Capitation Arrangements

Capitation arrangements should be structured to ensure that participating providers share financial risk at every level. For example, subcapitated specialists should have risk pools so that primary care physicians and specialists all are at risk for their respective colleagues' behavior. When structured this way, capitation contracting avoids price-fixing. Even individually capitated physicians, if the system is combined with other controls or incentives (for example, risk pools), may provide sufficient evidence of financial integration.

Fee-for-Service Contracting

Fee-for-service contracting poses the greatest risk of violating the antitrust laws. Several mechanisms can reduce (but not eliminate) this risk.

The Messenger Model
Antitrust risk is lessened when the network or IDS provides an agent (the messenger) who collects individual fee schedules from the individual participating

providers. This agent (who must not be a provider) is then the conduit for price negotiations between a particular payer and all the providers. The FTC has indicated approval so long as the messenger takes offers and counteroffers until there are a sufficient number of providers for a panel, but the messenger has *no* power to bind any of the providers and does not actually negotiate price. The network or IDS itself serves an administrative function thereafter by administering claims and performing utilization review functions. Although the messenger model is unwieldy and often creates logistical problems, its benefit is that it avoids any suggestion that the participating providers have jointly negotiated a fee schedule.

Payer Withholds

In this situation, the provider-controlled IDS engages the services of a third party to collect information from the providers and to develop a fee schedule. The IDS contracts with a payer and the payer pays a percentage (for example, 80 percent) of the amount provided in the fee schedule for every health procedure or encounter. The remainder is withheld by the payer and released at the end of the year *if* the IDS meets certain cost containment targets. The IDS then distributes the earned withhold amount to its providers on a predetermined sharing basis. This mechanism creates substantial risk sharing unless the withhold amount is not significant.

IDS Risk Withholds

Here the payer pays the entire fee negotiated in the fee schedule to the IDS and the IDS establishes a percentage withhold pool. The IDS sets up budgets and measure its providers' performance against these budgets. This method may promote a certain degree of cost containment; however, individual providers have little incentive to involve themselves in their colleagues' overutilization because overutilization increases the fees paid by the payer to the IDS and, therefore, increases the pool for the underutilizers to share.

The Black Box Approach

Here the third-party payer offers a fee schedule entirely independent from the IDS, after obtaining the necessary information from IDS providers. The IDS provider-based board simply accepts or rejects the fee schedule offered and makes no changes. This system avoids antitrust challenge of provider price-fixing, but does not promote cost containment goals or risk sharing. However, if providers are willing to relinquish control of pricing to the third-party payer's offer, fee-for-service pricing may be pursued in this manner with relatively little risk.

Most Favored Nation Clauses

Where payers impose a contractual term, requiring that the seller charge the payer no more than the lowest price that the seller charges any other payer (a most favored nation clause, or an MFN clause), both sellers and competing payers may be disadvantaged in seeking new and more attractive arrangements. However, in some court cases, MFN clauses have been sustained as procompetitive. Several state attorneys general have undertaken investigations of MFN situations where the payer has a significant market share. Some state legislatures have acted to prohibit MFN clauses in insurance policies.

Market Share/Market Power

A joint venture that includes an overly large share of the providers in the relevant market may have market power and be able, acting either by itself or with others, to raise prices or lower output. To determine if there could be a monopolization issue, the hospital should identify the geographic and product markets in which the venture operates. The term *geographic market* refers to the area where patients actually go for care and where they may practicably turn for it. Geographic markets are determined on a service-by-service basis. The term *product market* refers to those products or services that are reasonably interchangeable by consumers for the same purpose. The DOJ and the FTC use price increases as the test: If the price were to rise by a small amount, and not on simply a temporary basis, would this cause buyers to purchase a different product or service as a substitute? If so, are these additional products or services in the product market? Of course, an IDS may participate in more than one geographic or product market.

Exclusive Arrangements

To control the cost of providing health care services, payers frequently contract selectively with providers, excluding those hospitals, physicians, and others that are less efficient than their peers. If a network is to maintain or improve its efficiency, it will want to preserve its ability to exclude providers even after they have been admitted, by either expelling them or refusing to renew contracts. The disappointed hospital or physician may claim that the exclusion constitutes a group boycott or another form of illegal conduct. Enforcement agencies and courts recognize that selective contracting can have procompetitive effects. When some providers are excluded, they have an incentive to form a competing network or to contract individually with payers who seek to create their own provider panels. In fact, the FTC feels overinclusiveness raises far more substantial competitive concerns.

On the other hand, an IDS may face antitrust scrutiny if it fails to establish objective criteria for membership or if it ignores its own standards for membership when rejecting another provider's application. If providers are excluded solely because of pressure from competing providers and the IDS is unable to show any plausible efficiencies or procompetitive justifications for the exclusion, the risk of antitrust liability arises.

Generally, agreements between managed care payers and providers that limit or exclude referrals or other noncontracting provider involvement in the network usually avoid liability because of both the absence of market power and the procompetitive effects of such limitations. When some managed care payers require the contracting provider to refer patients within the contracted provider panel, this does not necessarily mean an illegal boycott has occurred. Courts have refused to undo such contracts just because a disappointed competitor also wanted the contract. This result is not unlawful and providers should not confuse an agreement to boycott with one to buy and sell services.

The Corporate Practice of Medicine Issue

In one IDS model, the foundation, a high degree of economic and operational integration is common. The foundation normally holds managed care contracts, bills and collects in its own name for services, and owns the patient medical records and accounts receivable. Such levels of integration are difficult to achieve in those states that recognize and enforce the corporate practice of medicine doctrine. One integration limitation found in states with corporate practice of medicine prohibitions is that the foundation cannot employ physicians directly but, rather, must contract independently with a physician group. Also, states that recognize the doctrine usually will not permit the direct splitting of professional services fees with nonprofessionals or the relinquishing of control by physicians over patient medical records, limiting to some degree the fuller integration possible in other states.

When structuring an IDS that has a hospital sponsor, it is important always to be aware that utilization of the various business forms and contractual arrangements available under various state laws to avoid conflict with the corporate practice of medicine doctrine may nevertheless result in conflicts with other key legal issues discussed in this handbook. The key legal issues that most frequently require balancing are tax exemption, Medicare fraud and abuse, and self-referral. For example, a nonprofit hospital's participation in the ownership of a medical services organization (MSO) (which might help solve the problem of the corporate practice of medicine doctrine) may result in the realization of unrelated business income by the hospital, which, if sufficient in amount, could jeopardize its federal tax-exempt status.

The funding of the various entities utilized by nonprofit hospitals to deal with the corporate practice of medicine doctrine may result in private benefit to the physicians who may be joint owners with the hospital in such enterprises, thereby further jeopardizing the hospital's federal tax exemption. Care also must be taken to avoid possible private-benefit consequences where state corporate practice of medicine doctrines permit limited direct employment of physicians. Further, both nonprofit hospitals and for-profit hospitals must be mindful of the illegal remuneration provisions of the federal Medicare/Medicaid fraud and abuse statutes in funding and compensating the various entities and physician arrangements utilized to avoid the doctrine's reach.

In addition to the financial relationship between an IDS and its physicians, the corporate practice of medicine doctrine also may affect the manner in which the IDS contracts with certain users of health care services. For example, some state HMO statutes require that HMOs contract for the delivery of health care services only with persons or entities licensed to provide those services. The doctrine also may limit the ability of an IDS to implement utilization review (UR) or utilization management of its physicians' services if such review, under state law, would be considered interference with the physician–patient relationship or a physician's independent control over medical decisions. The nature and extent of the UR activity will be important in determining application of the doctrine.

Because in some states a violation of the doctrine can lead to criminal or civil penalties and to physician discipline, including reprimand or license suspension or revocation, the effect of the doctrine on any given IDS should be reviewed carefully. The potential severity of penalties under state law must be balanced against the state's enforcement stance and the nature of any existing authority in the state in determining what level or levels of integration may be acceptable.

Another option in structuring an IDS may be to differentiate between different types of medical services. Some states treat the traditional hospital-based specialties (such as pathology, radiology, and anesthesiology) differently under the corporate practice of medicine doctrine. Thus, it may be possible to structure a system in such a way that some specialists are employed by the IDS (which bills for their services), while others are kept in a separate entity outside the IDS.

Where it is not possible to bring the physician component directly into the IDS, physicians must organize outside the IDS and contract with the IDS for the rendition of medical services. Normally, these are independent contractor arrangements in which the physician component maintains complete control over all medical decisions and retains all fees for professional services. One way to link the physicians in the contract service group to the IDS is to organize the IDS with joint ownership between the group (or the individual physicians) and the hospital.

Another integration link available in states following the corporate practice of medicine doctrine is the provision of various management services by the IDS to the physician group, such as billing and collection, accounting, record maintenance, marketing, and other administrative services. Under such a contractual arrangement, the IDS controls the business operations on behalf of the physician group and the physicians themselves merely perform the medical services. The IDS should charge the physician group a fair market value fee for the various administrative services it provides.

When separate entities are used and the IDS is linked together by contractual arrangements, a greater level of integration also can be achieved through overlapping memberships on boards of directors, advisory boards, and similar vehicles, where permitted. The use of coordinated board memberships can allow an IDS to attain a high degree of integration with its separate medical group, even where the corporate practice of medicine doctrine still exists.

The actual degree of ownership and control exercised by the system may vary. In some states following the corporate practice of medicine doctrine, an entity offering medical services may be owned by a nonphysician entity or have nonphysician directors if limitations are placed on lay control over medical judgments and fees for medical services. To satisfy these limitations, the following characteristics should be expressed in the IDS's organizational documents:

- Physicians control medical decisions including diagnosis and treatment.
- Physicians set and retain fees for medical services.
- Physicians maintain all patient records.
- Physicians maintain malpractice insurance responsibility.
- Physicians control their relationships with patients, including confidentiality and enforcement of covenants not to compete.

In sum, if the sponsor of an IDS is sufficiently flexible and imaginative, some or all of these approaches should permit some level of system integration with its physicians despite the active status of the corporate practice of medicine doctrine in the state.

Tax Exemption and Other Tax Issues

A corporation organized and operated exclusively for religious, charitable, scientific, literary, or educational purposes or testing for public safety may qualify for tax-exempt status under Section 501(c)(3) of the Internal Revenue Code. Two types of Section 501(c)(3) tax-exempt status exist: stand-alone and integral part.

The IRS has long recognized the promotion of health as a charitable purpose within the meaning of Section 501(c)(3). A hospital satisfies this purpose by serving the community in operating an emergency room open to all persons regardless of ability to pay, and providing hospital care for all persons in the community able to pay the cost either directly or through third-party reimbursement (such as private health insurance or public programs such as Medicare or Medicaid). Organizations that do not directly provide medical care also may promote the health of the community. For an IDS to achieve tax-exempt status, its structure and particular characteristics will have to meet the IRS's ever-increasing scrutiny. A determination letter should be obtained by counsel, unless the IDS is a mirror image of one the IRS has approved. It is not enough to be organized for tax-exempt purposes; the IDS's operations also must implement the IRS approved structure.

In 1993 and 1994, the IRS issued five tax-exempt determination letters in connection with the formation of IDSs.[9] In these rulings, the IRS required that the IDS have not more than 20 percent of the members of the board of directors be "financially interested" persons. These included employees (and perhaps former employees) and physicians currently or formerly employed or compensated by the hospital or the physician's clinic in the case. The 20 percent rule extended to IDS quorum and committee requirements; however, committees that consider the clinical or professional service aspects of the IDS could contain unlimited physician representation, but, committees created to consider physician compensation decisions could not include physician representatives who have a direct financial interest in the outcome of the decision.

The 20 percent rule is particularly problematic in the formation of most IDSs given the practical need to provide the physicians and the hospital with an equal share in governance to induce them to work together in a viable partnership. In its 1996 CPE (continuing professional education) textbook,[10] the IRS modified the 20 percent rule to exclude IDS and hospital administrative employees (and former employees); however, the rule is still applied to any physician currently or formerly employed by or with a financial link to the IDS.

When an IDS purchases one or more existing medical practices, the purchase price must be less than or equal to fair market value with proper allocations to intangible as well as tangible assets. Fair market value has been refined over time to "require" independent appraisals and arm's-length negotiations, and other details that hospitals should review with counsel.

The following checklist includes features that the IRS's 1996 CPE textbook identifies as showing that an IDS benefits the community:

1. Integration of all medical functions and records of each IDS patient, which may eliminate duplicate tests, procedures and treatments and result in greater efficiency and reduced cost to the public
2. Increase in accessibility to Medicare/Medicaid and charity patients
3. An open medical staff
4. An emergency room open to the public in which care is provided to all patients regardless of their ability pay
5. Service to all patients able to pay for care, including Medicare and Medicaid patients, together with:
   - A specific Medicare/Medicaid policy including access to all covered inpatient, outpatient and diagnostic services that are available to non-Medicare/Medicaid patients

- A willingness to enter into and pursue good faith negotiations with its state's Medicaid agency in an effort to obtain any available Medicaid contracts
- Participation in Medicaid fee-for-service arrangements at clinic locations (as opposed to merely serving Medicaid patients enrolled in managed care plans)

6. An agreement for professional services requiring physicians to:
   - Refrain from discriminating against individual patients based on ability to pay at the IDS's hospitals or clinic sites
   - Treat patients seeking urgent care at any IDS site without regard to ability to pay
   - Provide coverage in hospital emergency rooms and to render care therein without regard to the patient's ability to pay

7. The provision of research and education in the areas of primary and specialty care (including participation in internship or residency programs with an accredited medical school) and general health education programs for the public

8. An independent community board form of corporate governance

9. A charity care budget

10. Arm's length contract negotiations with physician groups selling their practices, and objectively determined compensation for physicians

The IRS also is concerned about how physician groups' financial relationships with a tax-exempt IDS can be protected against inappropriate favoritism or enrichment of these physicians. Necessary safeguards include:

- Medical group's compensation that is both reasonable and comparable to payment arrangements adopted by other medical groups of similar size and composition (by specialty) *net* of overhead now borne by the IDS.
- Independence of the IDS compensation committee and board decisions from interested physicians.
- Absence of any other arrangements suggestive of dividend-like sharing of charitable assets.

One fundamental concern for a tax-exempt hospital working with an IDS is whether acquisition of physician practices by the IDS or IDS operations will jeopardize the IDS's tax-exempt status (if it has one) or impair the hospital's. As most hospital executives are aware, the tax-exempt organization's net earnings cannot be used for the benefit of any private individual with an "inside" relationship to the organization. *Insiders* are individuals (such as directors, trustees, officers, major donors, or members of a hospital medical staff) whose relationship with an organization offers them an opportunity to make use of its income or assets for personal gain. The hospital must function as a public charity serving a public interest, not a private interest. How substantial the private benefit is will be measured in terms

of the overall public benefit conferred by the hospital's activity. These requirements must be addressed in the development and operation of an IDS (tax-
exempt or taxable) if it is capitalized by a tax-exempt hospital.

Application to Practice Acquisition Scenarios

Key tax-exemption issues for an IDS include the valuation of acquired practices, compensation to providers, recruitment and retention incentives, and
compliance with fraud and abuse laws.

Practice Valuation

To protect against private-benefit challenges, an IDS formed, in whole or
in part, with tax-exempt hospital funds must ensure that it purchases physician practices at fair market value. The IRS defines *fair market value* as
the price at which a willing purchaser and a willing seller agree, neither
being under any compulsion to buy or sell and both having reasonable
knowledge of the relevant facts. To evidence the fairness of the purchase
price offered to a physician, a valuation prepared by an independent, qualified valuation firm should be obtained. The valuation of the practice should
include:

- An executive summary
- A review of the nature of the business and history of the enterprise
- The economic outlook in general and that of the specific industry in
  particular
- The book value of the stock and hard assets and the financial condition
  of the business
- The earning capacity of the business
- The dividend-paying capacity of the business
- The estimated value of the intangible assets
- A description of the subject assets
- A discussion of comparable enterprises and their market value, where
  applicable

The IRS also will expect an analysis of the balance sheet, income statement, and financial performance ratios of the medical practice. The performance ratio analysis should focus on matters relating to liquidity, asset
management, debt management, and profitability. Negative factors that could
arise from this analysis include working capital position significantly below
industry average, an inappropriate credit policy, poor debt/equity ratios, and
poor profitability ratios. Valuations are not cheap, but the valuation process,
if properly done, will protect against challenges that the IDS bailed out a
weak practice resulting in private benefit to the selling physicians. It also

provides protection against challenges of illegal remuneration in the fraud and abuse context.

Compensation

Following acquisition, IDS compensation of its physicians or physician group (salaries and benefits) will be subject to close IRS review for reasonableness. The *IRS Audit Guidelines for Hospitals* highlight the relevant factors to be considered in establishing physician compensation:[11]

- Duties performed and amount of responsibility
- Time devoted to duties
- Special knowledge and experience
- Individual ability
- Previous training
- Compensation paid in prior years
- Working conditions
- Prevailing general economic conditions (including wage levels for work of similar scope and nature, price levels, and inflation)
- Living conditions in the particular locality

IDSs can look to several sources for physician compensation data including Medical Group Management Association's (MGMA's) annual Physician Compensation Survey.[12] The Graduate Medical Education National Advisory Committee of the Department of Health and Human Services, the AMA, state or local medical societies, and national trade associations for physician specialties are other likely sources, as are consulting firms and physician recruiting firms, practice management consulting firms, benefits and compensation firms, and the large accounting firms.

Some compensation variations, such as use of a cap on overall compensation, help distinguish a compensation for services arrangement from a joint venture or profit-sharing arrangement. However, incentive compensation raises the concern of a significant conflict between serving personal interests and serving the tax-exempt purpose of the organization. Accordingly, the IRS has approved incentive compensation arrangements, but only with the presence of certain safeguards. Generally, incentive compensation must serve a real and discernible business purpose, should have a cap, and when taken together with base salary and benefits, must be "reasonable" compensation for the services rendered. Incentive compensation also must not be a device to distribute profits of the IDS. In considering incentive arrangements, IDS executives should remember that providers can read and will follow incentive structures to maximize their income whether their activities result in harm or benefit to the IDS.

Recruitment and Retention

Efforts by tax-exempt organizations to facilitate physician–hospital integration may include incentives to recruit and retain physicians. Physician recruitment and retention incentives implicate federal tax-exempt laws, federal fraud and abuse statutes, federal and state laws addressing self-referral prohibitions, and other miscellaneous federal and state laws.

Different risks are posed to an institution's tax-exempt status depending on whether the physicians being recruited or retained are new to the region, will remain in private medical practices in their service area, or will provide full- or part-time services to the hospital. The IRS has indicated in Announcement 95-25 that the following techniques are acceptable for recruitment of a new physician into the hospital/IDS service area:[13]

- Providing start-up financial assistance
- Guaranteeing the physician's mortgage on a residence
- Payment of malpractice insurance premium for one year
- Payment by the hospital to the physician of a one-time bonus of up to $5,000
- Providing office space in a building owned by the hospital for three years at a below-market rent (after which the rental rate will be at fair market value)
- Reimbursement for professional liability "tail" coverage for the physician's former practice
- Guaranteeing private practice income for the first three years, based on regional or national surveys regarding income earned by physicians in the same specialty

All such arrangements must be predicated on established *community need* for the new physician, based on arm's-length negotiations, and set forth in a written agreement.

Fraud and Abuse Implications

Private-benefit issues often trigger parallel fraud and abuse concerns. As noted in a recent IRS bulletin: "Hospital F is located in City Z, a medium- to large-size metropolitan area. Because of its physician recruitment practices, Hospital F has been found guilty in a court of law of knowingly and willfully violating the Medicare and Medicaid Anti-kickback statute . . . for providing recruitment incentives that constituted payments for referrals. The activities resulting in the violations were substantial."[14] As a result, the IRS may revoke or deny tax exemption on top of the fraud and abuse penalties.

Similarly, medical practice valuation and provider compensation can raise Medicare/Medicaid fraud and abuse issues. The Office of the Inspector General's General Counsel's Office (OIG/GC) has asserted that certain assets ordinarily considered should not be included in assessing fair market value of a practice for purposes of the fraud and abuse laws. These include goodwill, going concern value, covenants not to compete, exclusive dealing provisions, and patient lists and patient records. The OIG/GC also have asserted that payments made by an employer to an employee for referrals cannot be included in a fair market value compensation determination because referrals are not "covered items or services" within the meaning of the fraud and abuse employment exception. Current legislative activity in this area suggests hospitals and IDSs should be very cautious in valuation and compensation matters.

The Hospital's Tax Status

Tax-exempt hospitals, or their affiliates, that participate in taxable joint ventures with nonexempt individuals or entities must be certain that their financial participation does not involve a private-benefit violation that would jeopardize the hospital's tax-exempt status. The IRS has held that a Section 501(c)(3) entity will not risk losing its exempt status so long as it does not make capital contributions to a taxable venture disproportionate to its share of the benefits to be derived. The IRS requires that there be evidence that the principal purpose of the venture genuinely is to benefit the community and not primarily to increase the hospital's market share by acquiring physician referrals. Contemporaneous documentation of community benefit is very important. Further, there must be true risk sharing by the non-tax-exempt participants.

If some or all of the taxable venture's activities do not relate to (support, promote) the participating tax-exempt hospital and its charitable purposes, the hospital (or tax-exempt participating subsidiary) will be subject to unrelated business income tax on that portion of the venture's distributions generated from activities that are unrelated to the exempt purposes.

There are two fundamental issues when a hospital considers using a taxable subsidiary for the development of an IDS:

1. Will owning 100 percent of the stock of a taxable corporation jeopardize the Section 501(c)(3) status of the hospital parent?
2. Will the taxable income of the subsidiary be taxable unrelated business income to the hospital parent?

To protect its tax-exempt status and avoid flow-through UBIT (unrelated business taxable income), the hospital should follow certain operating rules:

- Do not become actively involved in the day-to-day business affairs of its taxable subsidiary.

- Keep all transactions with the taxable entity at arm's length. This means charging the taxable entity fair market value fees for services the hospital provides, under written agreements.
- Allocate by usage the cost of any assets, facilities, or services shared between exempt and nonexempt affiliates.
- Keep clear the documentation of each organization as a genuinely separate corporations.

The extent of board of directors overlap between the tax-exempt hospital and its taxable subsidiary is only one factor the IRS will consider. Conservative advice recommends that no more than a minority of the officers and directors of the taxable subsidiary should also be officers or directors of the exempt parent. The more aggressive position allows substantial cross-directorships and cross-officerships, provided that the subsidiary's routine operations are free of the parent's involvement and that the subsidiary has a substantial and legitimate purpose. The IRS also will consider whether funding for the taxable affiliate's activities comes in whole or in part from an exempt hospital or affiliate through loan, guarantee, lease, or other contribution of property or cash.

Independent Contractor/Employee Issues

Recently, the IRS has been successful in arguing that despite the lack of control exercised by a hospital over how a physician practices medicine (that is, control over clinical and medical decisions), some arrangements with physicians constitute employer–employee arrangements. In doing so, the IRS has imposed substantial interest and penalties on the employer for its failure to withhold federal employment taxes from the reclassified employee's compensation. Typically, the IRS examinations have focused on hospital-based specialists (such as radiologists, anesthesiologists, and pathologists); however, they also will review other ongoing medical service arrangements.

The IRS's *Hospital Audit Guidelines* examines whether:[15]

- The physician has a private practice.
- The hospital pays straight wages to the physician.
- The hospital provides supplies and support staff.
- The hospital bills for the physician's services.
- The physician and the hospital divide the physician's fees on a percentage basis.
- The hospital regulates or otherwise has the right to control the physician.
- The physician is on duty at the hospital during specified hours.
- The physician's uniform bears the hospital's name or insignia.
- The hospital pays medical malpractice insurance premiums for the physician.

The *Hospital Audit Guidelines* also instructs examiners to consider the "twenty common-law factors" the IRS has traditionally used to make employment status determinations.[16] The common-law factors considered by agents include:

- The worker's training and compliance with instructions
- The level of integration of the worker's services into the business operations
- Whether services are rendered personally
- The hiring, supervision, and payment of assistants to the worker
- The continuity of the relationship
- Fixed hours of work
- Full-time commitment
- Performing the work on the employer's premises
- Order or sequence of work
- Oral or written reports
- Payment by hour, week, or month
- Payment of business and/or traveling expenses
- Furnishing of tools and materials
- Subsequent investment
- Realization of profit or loss
- Working for more than one firm at a time
- Making services available to the general public
- The rights to discharge or terminate the worker

An IRS Physician Issue Paper suggests that the following factors do not necessarily call for the conclusion that a physician is the hospital's employee:[17]

- Medical procedures performed in accordance with hospital protocols
- Internal hospital accreditation requirements for hospital privileges
- The use of hospital facilities
- The hospital's rights to terminate the physician's privileges for cause

The Physician Issue Paper identifies the following as the major factors typically present in a case in which the physician *is* an employee:[18]

- The institution reserves the right to specify the hours the physician must be present to perform medical services.
- The institution is entitled to fees collected for medical services rendered to patients.
- The institution bears the risk and expenses associated with delivery of medical care (for example, the cost of professional liability insurance, the provision of office space and supplies, and the furnishing of business support staff such as secretaries and transcriptionists).

Tax-Exempt Financing

There are tax-exempt financing considerations that are affected by hospital affiliations in IDS structures. Use of tax-exempt bond proceeds by a Section 501(c)(3) organization in an unrelated trade or business may cause the bonds to lose their tax-exempt status and trigger a default under bond documents. Other risks to tax-exempt financing include use of funds in a manner that could increase the risk of private benefit, such as using a for-profit manager for the tax-exempt facility or compensating the manager on the basis of the profits from the facility. There are special IRS "safe harbor" guidelines for management and service contracts involving use of property financed with tax-exempt bonds that should be carefully reviewed with legal counsel.

Summary of Tax Exemption Issues

Given the advantages of tax-exempt status under Section 501(c)(3) (including exemption from federal income tax, ability to receive tax-deductible contributions, ability to receive grants, possible exemption from state and local taxes, access to tax-exempt bond financing), and the fact that a substantial number of hospitals and other facility providers are tax-exempt entities, consideration of the particular organizational and operational requirements of tax-exempt organizations will be important in structuring many IDSs. In particular, the requirements for obtaining tax-exempt status, the tax-exemption implications of physician practice acquisitions, compensation issues after formation, and physician recruitment and retention all are areas that will be important in the formation of a tax-exempt IDS. Moreover, the use of particular forms of integration, such as joint ventures and taxable subsidiary corporations, is prevalent and important enough that significant attention should be paid to their particular advantages and disadvantages. Finally, because tax-exempt financing may be important as a unique and fruitful financing vehicle for the formation and operation of an IDS, recognition of the highly technical aspects governing such financing and the use of tax-exempt bond proceeds will prove necessary.

Pension and Other Benefits

Generally, two key benefit law concepts may interact within the most commonly proposed structures for an IDS, resulting in significant limitations on the range and amounts of benefits that may be made available to various groups of IDS employees. These concepts are nondiscrimination and aggregation for testing purposes of otherwise separate organizations. To preserve the favorable tax treatment for employee benefits, certain "nondiscrimination" tests must be satisfied. These tests focus on the treatment of an entity's non–highly compensated employees as compared to the highly compensated employees, known as the "prohibited group." Many important defined benefit or defined contribution pension plans favored by businesses are affected by this provision. The second key issue is whether entities that are related by common ownership or control, or in some cases on the basis of services provided, must be treated as a single employer for benefits purposes.

Each of the federal statutory sections relating to fringe benefit plans contains a separate set of nondiscrimination tests that must be passed to preserve favorable tax treatment for that particular benefit. Although it is not possible in this handbook to provide a specific overview of the nondiscrimination rules applicable to each of the various types of benefit plans, it is safe to say that all such tests are intended to prevent employee benefit plans from discriminating in favor of highly compensated participants as to either eligibility to participate or benefits provided. Failure of an employee benefit plan to satisfy both types of tests will cause the plan to lose its tax-favored status, at least with respect to the highly compensated group, causing the value of the benefits to become taxable income.

A general rule of thumb is that if the plan fails to benefit at least 70 percent of the non–highly compensated employees, the employer may have a problem satisfying the eligibility test. If the total number of employees against which the 70 percent rule is applied becomes larger as a result of aggregation under the affiliated service group rules, satisfying the eligibility or coverage tests may become increasingly difficult. The benefits tests analyze the actual level of benefits to which those individuals are entitled. Generally, the benefits tests require that the level of benefits provided to the non–highly compensated group, when compared to those provided to the highly compensated group, be very similar or, in some cases, identical. As a result, the ability to provide significantly richer benefits to only the highly compensated group (leaving aside the effect of integration with social security) is all but nonexistent in a qualified plan.

To prevent avoidance of the various nondiscrimination rules through the use of multiple entities, over the past 20 years Congress has enacted a series of complex statutory provisions under which separate legal entities must be aggregated and treated as a single employer for purposes of testing employee benefit plans for compliance with the various nondiscrimination rules discussed above. As a general matter, the more integrated the business and legal relationships between separate legal entitles, the more likely the entities will be required to be aggregated under these provisions.

There are five separate aggregation rules, each of which needs to be considered with counsel in evaluating whether the employees of separate legal entities must be aggregated for purposes of applying the various nondiscrimination requirements applicable to employee benefit programs. Generally, the five aggregation rules cover:

1. Employees of a "controlled group" of corporations
2. Employees of trades or businesses under common control
3. Employees of an "affiliated service group"
4. Certain "leased employees"
5. Other circumstances as the Secretary of Treasury may prescribe

The various forms of IDSs and arrangements among the IDS participants usually raise one or more of these aggregation rules.

The two controlled group rules are fairly mechanical to apply, because they are based on ownership of an entity. The affiliated service group rules and the leased employee rules are substantially more complex. For example, if the principal business of an organization is the performance of management functions for one other organization on a regular and continuing basis, the organization performing the management functions and the other organization may be treated as an affiliated service group, and their employees treated as employed by a single employer for purposes of the various nondiscrimination rules. Currently, there are no proposed or final regulations that provide further guidance as to how to apply the management functions test under the affiliated service group rules.

Similarly, application of the leased employees rules can result in individuals who are not traditional employees being treated as employees of the organization that receives their services. The key elements of the rule are:

- The nonemployee must provide services on substantially a full-time basis for at least one year.
- The services must be provided pursuant to an agreement between the recipient and another person (the leasing organization).
- The services performed must be of a type historically performed, in the business field of the recipient, by employees.

Employee leasing arrangements are not uncommon in the health and hospital industry. When physicians enter into participation agreements with preferred provider organizations (PPOs) and professional service agreements with insurance companies and other payers who contract with the PPO, this usually does not raise significant employee benefit concerns, because the relationship is contractual, not ownership or leasing. The situation could be different if the PPO were owned by the participating physicians.

An independent practice association (IPA) would not seem to raise significant employee benefit issues. However, where the services are provided on a capitated basis and risk sharing occurs, the IPA may be viewed as a joint venture among the contracting physicians and trigger the affiliated service group rules. The same issue may arise if the IPA provides management services to its members.

A clinic without walls form of integrated group practice may operate each clinic as a separate profit center or the operations of the various clinics may be combined. Such arrangements generally involve a single legal entity. Therefore, employee benefit issues generally will be limited to nondiscrimination compliance. However, where separate entities are maintained, they generally will have to be aggregated for employee benefit testing purposes. Many integrated medical groups involve complex business relationships among multiple entities, including professional service entities, management and administration entities, and separate entities holding real estate or equipment used by the groups. Generally, these separate entities will have to be aggregated for employee benefit purposes. When the business operations of a medical group are segregated into a separate MSO, and nonprofessionals hold equity interests in, or otherwise participate in, the governance of a practice, the MSO and the professional service entities will be aggregated for employee benefit purposes, particularly where the professionals have an equity interest in the MSO. MSOs also may be formed to service unrelated clinics, medical groups, or other practice entities. Whether the MSO will be aggregated with any of those entities depends on a detailed review of each case.

Another common situation involves a hospital with control over an IDS operating a new affiliated legal entity (a clinic, for example) that provides noninpatient medical services and hires physicians as either employees or independent contractors. The employees of the hospital and the clinic (as well as the employees of all other related entities) will be treated as employees of a single employer for most employee benefit purposes. If the clinic contracts with a medical group, the issue is whether the employees of the medical group (including the physicians) must be aggregated with the clinic and the hospital. If the clinic purchases the assets of the medical group and hires its employees to provide staff and administrative services to the medical group, the medical group would likely still have to cover such employees in its plans under the employee leasing rules. Furthermore, even if the services are provided by new employees, a leased employee issue could arise if the services are of a type historically performed by employees.

Similarly, if the medical group is compensated on a profit-sharing, rather than fixed-fee basis, the physicians could be deemed to be joint venture participants with the hospital and partners in the clinic. This would result in the medical group being included in an affiliated service group with the clinic and the hospital.

In the physician–hospital organization (PHO) structure, the PHO contracts with the hospital and the physicians to provide such services as may be required under its managed care service contracts. The aggregation issues raised by this structure are similar to those raised by the clinic model discussed above.

When integration of the hospital and physician service is accomplished by the hospital's management of the medical group, whether the medical group must be aggregated with the MSO depends on whether the affiliate service group or leasing rules apply and whether the medical group has an ownership interest in the MSO.

Insurance Licensure

An IDS usually offers the combined service of physicians, hospital(s), and other health care providers to payers. State law may require the IDS to obtain an insurance or HMO license if the IDS intends to contract directly with self-insured employers on a capitated basis or as a result of arrangements the IDS may establish with the third-party payer. Though IRS rulings suggest that an organization's direct provision of services for a fixed monthly rate is not an insurance function, many states take the position that only HMOs can agree to accept capitated payments.

The so-called center for excellence concept in which payers seek one packaged rate or a global fee for certain kinds of services (such as transplants and deliveries) is becoming increasingly popular. An argument can be made that these arrangements generally do not raise insurance licensure issues because they are essentially packaged fee-for-service compensation arrangements and do not involve the characteristics of insurance risk or an HMO. States vary on how they view these arrangements.

Some states assert that an organization that arranges services paid by capitation is a health plan under state HMO law, an insurance company, or both. Clearly, an HMO may contract with a group of physicians (perhaps an IPA) on a capitated basis. Whether that group of physicians may agree to provide (or arrange to provide) other health care services, such as hospital services, without obtaining its own HMO or insurance license is determined by state law. Some HMO laws may not authorize subcontracts to provide or arrange for comprehensive health care services, such as mental health, vision, or dental services, when paid by capitation. Some states also require licensure for independent utilization review or other administrative activities conducted on behalf of a payer or plan.

To solve the problem, an unlicensed IDS could limit providers' capitation to services under their direct control. Hospitals and all other providers not under direct control of the IDS would separately agree to capitation payments for their services. These arrangements, however, may compromise the desired full financial integration and risk sharing of the affiliated IDS providers.

A second approach would be a dollar limit, or cap, on the providers' assumption of risk, giving beneficiaries some regulatory relief if the provider group fails. The payer could be required to retain the risk for such services as emergency care or out-of-area services. Nevertheless, this type of arrangement may still be considered to be in violation of state insurance laws on prepayment and health plan features.

Third, the IDS could provide significant financial incentives in providers' compensation, short of financial risk. This approach may avoid insurance laws but may not be appealing to employers or other third-party payers.

Fourth, the IDS could seek regulatory or legislative clarification to allow capitated arrangements without HMO licensure. Whether the federal ERISA laws already govern in this area is still an open question.

Fraud and Abuse

The fraud and abuse or antikickback sections of the Social Security Act provide criminal penalties for individuals or entities that knowingly and willfully offer, pay, solicit, or receive remuneration in order to induce referrals of business reimbursed under the Medicare or state (Medicaid) health care programs.[19] Civil sanctions include exclusion of providers from participation in these programs. Substantial administrative penalties may also be imposed. Recently, private parties have successfully alleged violation of the antikickback laws to avoid enforcement of their contractual arrangements or to declare a transaction invalid.

The law covers not only remuneration to induce referrals of patients, but any remuneration intended to induce the purchasing, leasing, ordering, or arranging of any good, facility, service, or item paid for by Medicare or state health care programs. Because the wording of the law is so broad, safe harbor regulations describing those transactions that are not subject to prosecution or program exclusion have been issued by the OIG.

An arrangement that is not within a safe harbor does not necessarily constitute a clear statutory violation. For example, if a hospital funds the organization and initial operations of an affiliated IDS outside a safe harbor, the risk of violation may be low depending on whether (1) any aspect of the funding is based on anticipated referrals from the IDS to the hospital as a result of the establishment of the IDS, (2) establishment of the IDS is anticipated to alter existing referral patterns, and (3) the other economic transactions between the IDS and the hospital, or between the IDS and its physicians, support the intent of the antikickback statute.

The Safe Harbors

Because of the broad language of the fraud and abuse statute, in 1987 Congress directed the Office of Inspector General (OIG) of the Department of Health and Human Services to adopt "safe harbors" for activities and transactions that will be deemed not to violate the law.

Investment Interest

Ownership of an MSO providing administrative and management support services only, without contact with patients, generally will not violate the antikickback statute. However, an IDS, almost by definition, is engaged in providing health care services to patients. Its ownership structure may tend to affect the system's volume of business, thereby implicating the antikickback statute. The OIG investment interest safe harbor for small entities gives protection if no more than 40 percent of the investment interests are held by investors who can generate business or provide services to the entity, and if other requirements are met. A rural safe harbor allows individuals or entities who refer business to be owners if 75 percent of the patients served by the entity live in the rural area.

Personal Service and Management Contracts

The management services agreement of an MSO should meet the personal services and management contracts safe harbors. A written agreement of at least one year's length must specify an aggregate, fair market payment not based on the volume or value of referred business and the services covered; if part-time, the schedule of service intervals, their precise length, and the exact charge for such intervals must be included. No additional value for location or convenience to sources of Medicare/Medicaid business can affect compensation. Even in the case of an IDS, this safe harbor should be readily available. If a variety of services are provided, such as billing and collection, group insurance, managed care contracting, and so on, each service fee should be based on fair value; and a single fee charged for several services should be commensurate with the aggregated fair value of each service. Providers and IDSs must be able to document the basis for fair market value, and should research the range and type of compensation charged for those services in the community.

Rental Agreements

If an IDS or MSO leases office space or equipment from or to providers, it should follow the rental safe harbor, which follows the same basic regulatory points as the personal services safe harbor. An appraisal of the fair rental value of the premises will make compliance easier and also avoid disputes between the parties as to whether the rental is fair. The value of the site cannot take into consideration how close it may be to referral sources. With respect to equipment rentals, a similar process might be followed, if not cost prohibitive.

Employees

An employee safe harbor covers payments made by an employer to an employee who has a genuine (bona fide) employment relationship with the employer. Congress has been reviewing whether some employee arrangements for bonuses in obtaining referrals should be considered unlawful. Written employment agreements for IDS or MSO employees are desirable for purposes of obtaining the benefit of this safe harbor. Note that the definition of "employee" for purposes of this safe harbor may differ from the definition for IRS or state unemployment or worker compensation purposes.

Practice Acquisition

The practice acquisition safe harbor only protects sales between practitioners, not IDS or MSO purchases of physician practices. Though there has been a great deal of public debate on this topic, IDS and MSO purchases should follow the terms of the safe harbor, or come as close as possible to the safe harbor, to stay within the intent of the statute. The OIG's senior counsel has publicly acknowledged that physician practice acquisitions, whether by a practitioner, IDS, or MSO, predicated on fair market value and not taking into account any value of referrals are permissible. Therefore, when an IDS or an MSO purchases physician practices, it should obtain a written opinion of an independent, expert appraisal firm that the acquisitions are at fair market value and do not attribute value to the referrals from the acquired practices to either the IDS, the MSO, or the affiliated hospital in order to reduce the risk for a violation of the antikickback statute by reason of the practice purchases.

Referral Services

The safe harbor for referral services should be reviewed if the IDS or MSO contemplates operating a referral service to handle incoming calls from prospective patients. A referral service may not exclude any person or entity that meets participation qualifications, which may be established according to the organization's own criteria. These criteria must be applied equally to all participants. The referral service must disclose to persons seeking referrals from the service how the group of participants is selected, how individual participants are chosen, whether a fee is paid, the relationship between the participant and the service, and any restrictions that would exclude a participant. Fees may not exceed the actual cost of operating the referral service. Although the referral service cannot dictate to the physician how services are to be furnished, the physician may be barred from the referral service if he or she is engaging in discriminatory pricing.

Group Purchasing and Discounts

The IDS or MSO may find that instituting a group purchasing program for the benefit of the participants in the organization is desirable. The group purchasing organization (GPO) safe harbor focuses primarily on fees that vendors might pay to an entity (such as the IDS or MSO to the extent that it acts as a GPO) for the privilege of securing its group-purchasing business. The discount safe harbor focuses primarily on tying the discount to a particular purchase and requires that the discount generally be provided at the time the transaction occurs.

OIG Fraud Alerts

The OIG periodically issues so-called "fraud alerts" about practices it considers improper. These alerts have included warnings on suspect joint ventures and on hospital incentives to physicians.

Joint Ventures

In 1989, the OIG issued a fraud alert on joint ventures that cautioned that joint ventures involving the following would be considered suspect:

- Investors as potential referral sources
- Physicians likely to be large referral sources who are provided an opportunity to purchase larger shares in the entity
- Physicians encouraged to refer to the entity or to divest their interest if referrals fall below an "acceptable" level
- An entity's tracking and distributing information regarding referral sources
- Physicians' divestiture upon retirement or other change in status linked to the ability to make referrals to the entity
- Extraordinary returns on an investment in comparison with the risk involved
- Physician investors "borrowing" the amount of the "investment" from the entity, paid by deductions from profit distributions

Hospital Incentives to Physicians

In 1992, the OIG issued another fraud alert on suspect incentives to recruit and retain physicians, highlighting:

- Payment of any sort of incentive by the hospital each time a physician refers a patient to the hospital
- Use of free or significantly discounted office space or equipment (in facilities usually located close to the hospital)
- Provision of free or significantly discounted billing, nursing, or other staff services
- Free training for a physician's office staff in areas such as management techniques, CPT coding, and laboratory techniques
- Guarantees that if the physician's income fails to reach a predetermined level, the hospital will supplement the remainder up to a certain amount

- Low-interest or interest-free loans, or loans that may be "forgiven" if a physician refers patients (or some number of patients) to the hospital
- Payment of the cost of a physician's travel and expenses for conferences
- Payment for a physician's continuing education courses
- Coverage under the hospital's group health insurance plans at an inappropriately low cost to the physician
- Payment for services (which may include consultations at the hospital) which require few, if any, substantive duties by the physician, or payment in excess of the fair market value of the services rendered

The Stark Prohibitions

The Stark laws significantly expanded the restrictions on physician referrals of Medicare and Medicaid patients. The broad Stark I and II physician self-referral prohibitions directly affect vertically-integrated IDSs because if a physician or an immediate family member has a "financial relationship" with the IDS, the physician may not refer a Medicare or Medicaid patient to that entity, and the entity may not submit a bill, for any of the following designated health services (DHSs) unless an "exception" exists:

- Clinical laboratory services
- Physical therapy services
- Occupational therapy services
- Radiology or other diagnostic services
- Radiation therapy services
- Durable medical equipment (DME)
- Parenteral and enteral nutrients, equipment, and supplies
- Prosthetics, orthotics, and prosthetic devices
- Home health services
- Outpatient prescription drugs
- Inpatient and outpatient hospital services

Prohibited Self-Referrals

Referrals include requests by a physician for an item or service; for a consultation with another physician and any test or procedure ordered, performed, or supervised by the consulting physician; and for (or establishment of) a plan of care, including a DHS. The following activities are not referrals provided they are furnished by, or under the supervision of, the pathologist, radiologist, or radiation oncologist, and are performed pursuant to a consultation requested by another physician:

- Requests by pathologists for clinical diagnostic laboratory tests or pathological examination services

- Requests by radiologists for diagnostic radiology services
- Requests by radiation oncologists for radiation therapy services

Financial relationships are (1) direct ownership or investment interests in the DHS entity, or indirect ownership (ownership through another entity that owns or invests in the entity) by the referring physician or an immediate family member of that physician, including through equity, debt, or other means; or (2) virtually any other type of compensation arrangement between the referring physician or an immediate family member of that physician and the DHS entity.

Compensation arrangements cover any remuneration directly or indirectly, overtly or covertly, in cash or in kind, between a physician (or an immediate family member) and a DHS entity, except:

- Forgiveness of amounts for inaccurate or mistakenly performed tests or procedures, or the correction of minor billing errors.
- Items, devices, or supplies used solely to collect, transport, process, or store specimens for the entity providing them; or to order or communicate the results of tests or procedures for that entity.
- Fee-for-service payments on behalf of a patient made by an insurer or self-insured plan to a physician for covered services when the physician does not have a contract with that insurer or plan. The amount must be preset, not in excess of fair market value, and not based, directly or indirectly, on the volume or value related to any referrals.

Stark Exceptions

The Stark I and II exceptions are written in statutes so there is *no gray area* between failing to fully qualify for an exception and actually violating the law. Plain and simple, if a physician or an immediate family member of that physician is deemed to have a "financial relationship" with a DHS entity, the physician is absolutely prohibited from referring a patient to that entity for a DHS and the entity is absolutely prohibited from submitting a bill for that service.

Group Practice Exception
One exception is for group practices and covers all DHSs personally provided by the referring physician or an individual directly supervised by the physician, other than DME, parenteral and enteral nutrients, and equipment and supplies (including infusion pumps). The difficult and changing issue has been the definition of *group practice.* The final regulations for Stark I (labs) suggest a very complicated process for determining a group practice. The features include centrality of location for the practice or the DHS; billing controlled by the physician, group, or billing company; a true legal form

for the practice; and a complex mathematical formula for overall physician participation by the group members. Required attestations about group practice participation have recently been delayed, due at least in part to confusion over these rules.

Ownership or Investment Exception

There is a narrow exception for in-network referrals by physicians who have ownership or investment interests in, or compensation arrangements with, certain Medicare HMOs, federally qualified HMOs, or other prepaid plans operating under a demonstration project. Congress also provided that ownership or investment interests in the following would not trigger the self-referral ban:

- Publicly traded securities and mutual funds, or a regulated investment company having total assets exceeding $75 million
- Hospitals in Puerto Rico
- A rural provider if "substantially all" of the DHSs are furnished to individuals residing in a rural area
- A hospital where the referring physician is authorized to perform services, provided that the ownership or investment relates to the hospital itself and not merely to a subdivision

Compensation Exception

Congress also decided that certain compensation arrangements would not trigger the self-referral ban. These include:

- *Rental of office space or equipment rental:* This exception follows the anti-kickback safe harbor. There must be a signed, written agreement of at least a year in length for no more space or equipment than is reasonable and necessary, and priced in advance at fair market value, without regard to the volume or value of any referrals or other business generated. The lease must be "commercially reasonable" even if no referrals were made.
- *Genuine employment relationships:* These are for identifiable services, at fair market value without regard to volume or value of any referrals, and commercially reasonable even if no referrals were made by the physician to the employer. IRS standards for employees are applied.
- *Personal service independent contractor arrangements:* These must be of at least a year's length, signed and in writing, for all specific services provided by the physician (or immediate family member) to the DHS entity. The aggregate services must not exceed what is reasonable and necessary for the legitimate business purposes of the arrangement, and must be set in advance at fair market value without regard to volume or value of any referrals or other business generated. Certain qualifying physician incentive plans are permitted if they may reduce or limit services.

- *Remuneration unrelated to the provision of a DHS:* Payments unrelated to furnishing health services are permitted.
- *Physician recruitment payments:* These may be made to induce a physician to relocate to the hospital's service area provided referrals to the hospital are not considered in calculating the recruitment payment.
- *Isolated transactions:* These are transactions such as the one-time sale of a property or a medical practice, if the price paid is fair market value and does not take into account referrals.

Hospital-Based Services

Hospitals may pay physician groups for DHSs that are inpatient hospital services provided by the group and billed by the hospital if (1) the arrangement began before December 19, 1989, and has continued in effect; (2) substantially all of the DHSs furnished to hospital patients are furnished by the group under the arrangement; and (3) the arrangement with the group is in writing and specifies services and compensation at fair market value without regard to volume or value of any referrals or other business generated between the parties. This latter point will be difficult for many hospitals to satisfy, since many such arrangements establish compensation on a per-procedure or per-visit basis.

Clinical Laboratory Services

The prohibitions also do not cover physician payments to a laboratory in exchange for the provision of clinical laboratory services, or to compensate the lab or another entity for other items or services furnished at a price consistent with fair market value.

Stark Reporting and Penalties

DHS entities must report to the Health Care Financing Administration (HCFA) the names and identification numbers of all physicians who have (either directly or through an immediate relative) an ownership or investment interest in the entity. Failure to comply with various reporting requirements can result in the imposition of a civil money penalty (CMP) of up to $10,000 a day.

The mandatory penalty for violation of the self-referral ban is a denial of payment for the DHS rendered in violation of the ban, or a refund of any amounts billed and collected for the DHS. The mandatory recapture of all gross revenues derived from impermissible referrals can be financially devastating even for the most fiscally sound facilities, and may even lead to bankruptcy.

The OIG also may impose a CMP (civil monetary penalty) of up to $15,000 for each DHS bill or claim that the person knew or should have known was rendered in violation of the self-referral ban. The OIG may seek a CMP of up to $100,000 on any physician or entity that enters into a circumvention scheme (such as a cross-referral arrangement) that the physician or entity knows or should know has a principal purpose of ensuring referrals which, if made directly by the physician to the entity, would violate the self-referral ban.

Any physician, hospital, or other entity subject to a CMP also may be assessed up to twice the amount claimed for each DHS violating the self-referral ban. In addition, they may be excluded from participation in the Medicare and Medicaid programs for several years. For any hospital, this exclusion would be the "death penalty." Enforcement efforts under the Stark laws conceivably could rely on automatic computer checks and cross-references among the multitude of physician and facility data already housed in computer databanks for the Medicare program.

Stark Issues Affecting the IDS

Every time an IDS contracts with a physician who is in a position to refer Medicare and Medicaid patients to the IDS for ancillary services that are included on the DHS list, a potential Stark problem arises. Where an IDS merely contracts with unrelated third parties for provision of a DHS, IDS physician referrals to those entities will not trigger the self-referral ban unless the physician has a separate financial relationship with the entity furnishing the services. However, where an IDS sets up a subsidiary to furnish a DHS, or where an IDS operates one or more DHSs as part of its own line of business, IDS physician referrals will be prohibited outright unless the IDS complies fully with the statutorily enumerated criteria under one of the Stark exceptions. Furthermore, referrals to and from an IDS for inpatient and outpatient services are subject to the self-referral ban. Therefore, physicians who have a financial relationship with an IDS or a hospital may not refer patients to these entities for a DHS unless the relationship between the physician and IDS or hospital clearly fits within an exception.

In the IDS formation stage, the exception for isolated transactions should insulate physician practice acquisitions where the transaction is commercially reasonable and the purchase price is consistent with fair market value and unrelated to the volume or value of referrals. OIG officials and proposed Stark regulations have stated that a truly isolated transaction must not include any extended financing by the selling physician or group, such as a note from the IDS as partial payment. Also, payments to entice physicians to relocate to the geographic area of the IDS hospital should be permitted under the exception for physician recruitment, where the physician is not required to make referrals to the hospital and the payments to the physician are unrelated to the volume or value of referrals.

Once an IDS is established, several exceptions are available to protect payments to physicians. Depending on whether the physician is employed by the IDS or independently contracted, the exceptions for bona fide employment relationships and personal service arrangements will be available where the payment to the physician is for identifiable services, consistent with fair market value, and unrelated to the volume or value of referrals; and the other exception-specific criteria discussed earlier also are satisfied. The exceptions for rental of office space or equipment rental also can protect those physician–IDS arrangements that satisfy the exception-specific criteria. It should be noted that the employment exception permits payment of productivity bonuses to employee physicians where the bonus is based on services personally performed by the physician. The exception for personal service arrangements specifically permits the use of withhold pools and capitation payments provided that there is "no intention to reduce or limit medically necessary services."

Finally, the exception for remuneration unrelated to the provision of a DHS permits payments to physicians for operating a utilization review or quality assessment program or serving as either a department head or in another administrative capacity. This exception also may protect hospital loans to physicians for certain integration activities, such as organizational costs.

Reimbursement and Payment Issues

Medicare payment issues raised by IDSs primarily center on limitations on who can bill for services. These limitations should be considered when structuring the IDS.

Incident-to Rules

Medicare generally requires medical professionals whose services are billed as "incident to a physician's services" to be under common employment with the physician. Medicare allows the physician to bill for nonphysician services incident to his or her services only if the nonphysician services are performed under his or her direct supervision. Medicare has interpreted this as requiring common employment. To bill for these nonphysician services, the physician must be actively involved in the patient's course of treatment, immediately available to the nonphysician when the service is being performed, and the service must be an expense to the physician's practice. Medicare also covers services or supplies incident to a physician's professional service when they are an integral, although incidental, part of the physician's diagnosis or treatment of an injury or illness.

Similar rules govern services in a physician-directed clinic or group association. In highly organized, departmentalized clinics, several physicians (not just one individual) may supervise. The ordering physician may not be the physician supervising the service. Services performed by therapists and other aides are covered even though they are performed in another department of the clinic, and supplies used in clinic treatment also are covered.

Auxiliary personnel services outside the clinic premises are covered only if performed under the *direct* supervision of a clinic physician. Ancillary staff providing incident-to services must be employed by the clinic or group association, and any physician in the group can bill for their services. Diagnostic X-ray services and other diagnostic tests must be furnished by a physician, or incident to a physician's service, to be covered by Medicare. These include basal metabolism readings, EEGs, EKGs, respiratory function tests, cardiac evaluations, allergy tests, physiological tests, and otologic examinations. To date, there is no national Medicare policy specifically addressing which types of arrangements for services of auxiliary personnel will meet the employment relationship requirement.

Reassignment

Medicare generally prohibits reassignment of benefits. This prohibition can significantly affect the structure of the IDS. An IDS must, therefore, fit within one of the following Medicare permitted payment assignment situations:

- From a physician employee to his or her employer if the employment arrangement requires assignment and the physician is recognized as an employee by IRS standards.
- From a physician to a facility (hospital, nursing home, and so on) if there is a written agreement with the physician under which only the facility can bill for the physician's services provided in the facility.
- From a physician to an organized health care delivery system that is paid for delivery of health care to individuals and groups of individuals, such as a medical group clinic that is paid to provide diagnostic or therapeutic medical services on an outpatient basis in quarters that it owns or leases. All services for patients of the clinic must be furnished within its physical premises unless the physician is a sole proprietor, partner, or employee.
- From a physician to a billing or collection service retained by the physician provided the fee for services is not related to the dollar amounts billed or actually collected. In this situation, the physician can direct how payments are handled and the agent acts only for the physician.

One problem related to reassignment is the difficulty of obtaining more than one physician identification number (PIN). If a physician has a PIN assigned through a clinic, he or she may be unable to obtain a PIN individually. A related problem arises because payment levels vary depending on type of provider and site of service. Some resource-based relative value scale (RBRVS) payments are established regardless of setting. Ultimately, managed care may make the setting and type of provider less or not at all relevant to payment levels.

Other Reimbursement Considerations

Other Medicare reimbursement rules may affect the IDS structure.

Funded Depreciation

Medicare restricts the use of funded depreciation to patient care–related purposes of the provider. Funded depreciation segregated accounts are used for acquisition of depreciable assets related to patient care. The funded depreciation must be readily marketable in investments to ensure the availability and conservation of the funds. Investment income not meeting this condition must be offset against allowable interest expense.

Cost Reimbursement

As of year-end 1995, Medicare cost-based reimbursement still included:

- Skilled nursing facilities
- Home health agencies
- Comprehensive outpatient rehabilitation facilities
- Exempt psychiatric and rehabilitation hospitals and distinct part units of hospitals
- Long-term hospitals (average length of stay greater than 25 days)
- Rural health clinics

Other Issues

Traditional Medicare concerns include allocation of overhead with the necessary separation of operations; related party elimination of reimbursement for profit; and cost reporting for a home office providing significant services to another entity that files a cost report. These issues may diminish to the extent Medicare moves away from cost-based reimbursement to a prospective payment system (PPS) and other managed care reimbursement mechanisms.

References

1. 15 U.S.C. § 1.
2. 15 U.S.C. § 2.
3. 15 U.S.C. § 13.

4. 15 U.S.C. § 18.

5. *See* 15 U.S.C. § 18a.

6. 15 U.S.C. § 45.

7. 457 U.S. 332 (1982).

8. *Statement of Antitrust Enforcement Policy in the Health Care Area* issued jointly by the Federal Trade Commission and the Department of Justice (Sept. 1993).

9. For a more detailed discussion of these rulings, *see Hospital-Affiliated Integrated Delivery Systems: Formation, Operation and Contracts Handbook.* American Academy of Healthcare Attorneys Practice Guide Series. Vol. 2 at 90 to 94 (1995).

10. Internal Revenue Service. *Continuing Professional Educational Exempt Organizations Technical Instruction Program Textbook.* 1996 edition. (IRS release Aug. 1995).

11. *IRS Audit Guidelines for Hospitals, Manual Transmittal* 7(10)69-38; *Exempt Organizations Guidelines Handbook* Section 331(1)(Mar. 27, 1992).

12. *See* MGMA Physician Compensation Survey. *Physician Advisory Newsletter*

13. IRS Announcement 92-25, Internal Revenue Bulletin 1995-14 (Apr. 3, 1995).

14. IRS Announcement 92-25.

15. *New Audit Guidelines* § 333.7; *See also,* Manual Transmittal 7(10)69-38 for *Exempt Organizations Examination Guidelines Handbook,* dated Mar. 27, 1992.

16. *New Audit Guidelines.*

17. *See* Daily Tax Rep. (BNA) Mar. 26, 1993, at L-1.

18. *See* Daily Tax Rep.

19. 42 U.S.C. § 1320a-7b.

Chapter 3

Operational Issues of Integrated Delivery Systems

In this chapter, several of the most common operational concerns of integrated delivery systems (IDSs) are reviewed in light of the legal issues introduced in earlier chapters.

Provider Selection and Exclusion Issues

Efforts to respond to managed care payer requirements often result in providers organizing into smaller and more tightly controlled groups, which can give rise to antitrust and other legal issues.

Antitrust Concerns

A managed care organization (MCO) is any organization that operates a managed care plan or contracts to be a participant in managed care plans, and includes payers who organize provider panels for plans, independent practice associations (IPAs), physician–hospital organizations (PHOs), or the various forms of IDSs. When a provider is excluded from an MCO, there are three possible complaints the MCO executive may have to handle, whether or not the facts support them:

1. *Group boycott:* Group boycott claims grow out of decisions to exclude some providers from participating in the MCO. These claims can be avoided or minimized by (1) insulating competing providers from making decisions about the provider during the selection, review, and termination processes; and (2) basing all participation decisions on articulated, objective criteria uniformly applied to all providers.
2. *Lack of access to an "essential facility":* Generally, there is no duty to help one's competitors, but an essential facility is one so important that others in the market cannot compete without it. Therefore, the facility

must be available to competitors, if practical, on a reasonable and non-discriminatory basis.

3. *Monopolization:* Because monopolization is the willful acquisition or maintenance of monopoly power, if an MCO has market power in any of the markets in which it or its component providers operate, it could face complaints. MCOs with large market shares are at risk if they have most favored nation and exclusivity provisions. Organizations with smaller market shares should avoid any step that looks like an attempt to acquire market power by unlawful means.

Group Boycott

The major risk from a true boycott is that the court could decide the action is absolutely, per se illegal without consideration of the positive features of the arrangement for high-quality care or efficiency in health services. An MCO could be accused of boycotting when it deals exclusively with certain physicians or hospital providers. The MCO could itself complain about a boycott if certain providers collectively refuse to deal with it and instead deal with some other organization. However, most MCOs will be able to show that they do not control enough business to meet the definition of dominant market power. In the health care field, the Supreme Court has decided that a 30 percent share of the relevant market is insufficient for a finding of dominant market power. The Court also has said that concerted refusals to deal might have a plausible justification based on enhanced efficiency or competition. For example, exclusion of physicians might be acceptable if the physicians' practice history suggests that they will not comply with cost containment standards.

An excluded provider is unlikely to prove an MCO's decision is illegal when the organization has a small share of the market where the MCO and provider operate. In this circumstance, the provider has sufficient opportunities to deal with other MCOs and insurers. Furthermore, even if the exclusion affects one provider, the issue is whether overall competition in the market is affected adversely. A refusal to deal with a class of providers, such as chiropractors or podiatrists, is therefore more likely to raise significant antitrust issues, because overall competition is more likely to be affected.

Group boycott claims have been made about the denial of hospital staff privileges, particularly where individual physicians have the right to veto the grant of privileges to another physician. However, small market share and lack of unique reasons for open access to a particular hospital have supported the hospital actions. The grant of exclusive privileges by a hospital to a physician or group of physicians also has been upheld where the policy was grounded in ensuring high-quality patient care and necessary hospital services. No formal hearing process is necessary if the exclusion is by either the medical staff bylaws or a contract between the practitioner and the hospital.

When an MCO panel votes on exclusion of providers, a critical factor is *who* makes the exclusion decisions. Sometimes the payer or a third party makes utilization review, quality assurance, or other decisions that may result in a provider exclusion. In those cases, absent highly unusual facts, the MCO generally will have no antitrust exposure. Furthermore, the Joint Policy Statement of the Federal Trade Commission/Department of Justice (FTC/DOJ) indicates greater concern with overinclusiveness than limited network panels.

There are arguments to defend against a group boycott challenge. First, a boycott must be "concerted action." If the decision to exclude is only one-sided (does not involve multiple parties), it is not illegal. For an MCO to obtain this protection, it must be a truly "integrated" joint venture and not simply a loose group of independent providers. The FTC asserts that integrated arrangements involve pooled capital and the sharing of "substantial" provider risk due to utilization or cost of health services. Also the criteria for excluding providers should be developed in advance, with appropriate input from physicians. Ultimate approval of the criteria should be made by a governing body not involved in developing them. Clearly, a non-provider-controlled MCO will have considerably less antitrust exposure than a provider-controlled MCO making these provider participation/exclusion decisions. An MCO that is not provider controlled may be considered simply a purchaser of services. If the organization is provider controlled, the question is the same as in a price-fixing analysis: Is the organization a true, integrated joint venture in which provider selection decisions are necessary to further its legitimate purposes? Courts have examined the nature and power of provider committees and provider board representation to determine whether the providers were authoritative or merely advisory to a non-provider-dominated decision-making body.

From an antitrust perspective, there may be nothing wrong with an organization negotiating with a provider in an arm's-length, good-faith manner, even when the result is exclusion of competing providers. Therefore, the second boycott defense is that the motive for the exclusive contract was based on legitimate and defensible reasons, such as cost containment or quality of care. However, when discussions start between the MCO and competing providers that may lead to exclusionary decisions, the line between permissible "communication" and impermissible "collaboration" may not be clear and hospital representatives should be very cautious.

The third defense against a boycott claim is that the market power effect is not sufficient to demonstrate real harm, such as preventing entry into the market by other managed care panels or alternative delivery systems.

Essential Facility

According to antitrust case law, an entity that controls a facility "essential" to its competitors may be guilty of monopolization if it refuses to allow them reasonable access to the essential facility and it is impractical or unreasonable to expect the competitors to duplicate the facility. Hospital staff privilege circumstances probably are not subject to this doctrine. However, a physician-dominated MCO that has significant market power through its payer contracts could be vulnerable. Under this doctrine, the essential physician organization could be the "facility," and could not unreasonably deny preferred provider status to a clearly qualified applicant. No case has yet determined that an MCO constitutes an essential facility.

Monopolization

An MCO with market power also raises concern if it requires its participating physicians to sign contracts that effectively bar them from participating in any other MCOs and if the other MCOs cannot recruit a sufficient provider panel in the area to be competitive. If an MCO were so ambitious as to obtain almost universal provider participation in its marketing area and demand exclusivity, the contractual requirement could constitute strong evidence of an anticompetitive intent to obstruct new MCO development in that market and therefore to monopolize. Once again, the market power of the plan or organization is at the heart of the question and a high percentage guarantees close scrutiny. However, an MCO and its participants may in any event continue to exclude incompetent providers.

Providers acting through the MCO may also engage in monopolization. When providers choose, for various reasons, not to contract with a payer, their decision *might* raise concerns if the providers have extensive market power and the payer could fail in the marketplace without the provider contract or if any provider had based its refusal on a previous agreement with other providers or with another payer. The first situation could easily arise in a one-hospital town or a small community with one dominant physician group.

Reducing Liability from Exclusion Decisions

If an organization has the following features, a good argument exists that it is a bona fide integrated joint venture and can survive group boycott challenges:

- Pooling of substantial capital among the participants
- Sharing of the risk of loss among the participants, as well as the potential for profit, through capitation contracts or withhold arrangements among the participating providers
- Utilization review protocols
- Joint marketing, claims administration, and billing and collection
- Competition for business with similar entities

If the MCO is provider controlled, it also should have objective membership criteria, including written objective standards for admission to and termination from the organization. Presumably, so long as the objective standards are not anticompetitive, courts will be less likely to reverse the organization's exclusionary decisions. The disadvantages to operating with objective criteria include:

- Application of objective criteria can be somewhat burdensome. Developing the statistical and other data to apply the criteria takes considerable time and effort.
- It is difficult to apply objective standards consistently. Making an exception for what seems like a good reason can erode the criteria altogether.
- Failure to adhere to standards places an unnecessary additional legal burden on the organization by giving an unhappy provider a claim for not following standards as well as for the exclusion.
- Objective standards may be inconsistent with the organization's business objectives. The organization may have a business need to deal with certain providers to the exclusion of others, no matter the adopted standards.

The MCO's business plan should set specific levels of provider participation, by geographic and specialty needs. Providers should not determine the substance of the business plan as it applies to competitors. The application and quality assurance process should be thorough and fair, with competitor participation only in carefully limited roles. The use of agreed-on practice parameters can streamline the peer review portion of the quality assurance process through physician consensus.

By not involving physicians directly in business plan elements affecting competing physicians, certain classes of practitioners (for example, podiatrists and chiropractors), and allied health professionals, the risk of challenge to exclusion decisions will be reduced. In multihospital MCOs, competing hospitals should not participate directly with each other in preparing the business plan.

Other Claims by Excluded Providers

In addition to antitrust claims, an excluded provider may assert provider protection provisions of the state insurance laws and other state common-law protections against an MCO's decision. If a state has adopted so-called any willing provider or antiexclusionary statutes and regulations, and if MCOs are subject to state insurance regulation, the state may require MCOs to give providers a fair opportunity to contract. Often states also have antidiscrimination laws aimed at one or more particular classes of providers, such as chiropractors, nurse practitioners, or podiatrists. Because these laws affect covered services under regulated health plans, it is disputed whether these laws require that membership be offered to willing or protected providers by unregulated MCOs (IPAs, broker PPOs, ERISA [Employment Retirement Income Security Act] self-insured employer plans, and so on).

The Health Care Quality Improvement Act (HCQIA)[1] provides immunity under certain conditions for peer review activities of "health care entities." The law applies to health maintenance organizations (HMOs) and group medical practices that provide health care services and follow a formal peer review process, including due process and a hearing on appeal of an adverse decision, for the purpose of furthering high-quality health care. Many MCOs do not actually provide health care services but, rather, contract with others for their provision. Therefore, the HCQIA protection will probably not be available to nonprovider MCOs. Also, the HCQIA immunity is only available for decisions based on competence or professional conduct.

Even with a fair review process, excluded providers may argue whether the exclusionary actions were taken in good faith. Organizers of an MCO should determine whether the benefits of HCQIA protection, including antitrust immunity and access to the data bank, outweigh its detriments, among which are mandatory reporting to the data bank for adverse credentialing decisions based on professional competence or conduct and complying with the requirement of statutorily defined full due process.

Managed Care and Health Care Information

Computerization of the patient medical record, reduction of administrative costs in health delivery, and broad accessibility to financial and outcomes data are essential to the managed care market today. To realize its potential, an MCO must process claims, obtain eligibility and benefits information, perform preauthorization procedures, coordinate benefits, and provide utilization and case management functions. The sharing of information within a health delivery system can raise significant concerns about confidentiality and control.

Obligations to Maintain Confidentiality

Physicians and hospitals are bound by professional codes of ethics to maintain patient confidentiality and safeguard against disclosure of records without patient consent. State statutes and licensure laws and federal conditions of participation for hospitals and other institutional providers require strict adherence to privacy standards. Some states (such as California) define the circumstances under which providers, employers, and third-party administrators may release individually identifiable health information to third parties. Many states impose confidentiality requirements on HMOs by statute or regulation, and several states have adopted the National Association of Insurance Commissioners model act, which imposes confidentiality obligations on insurance institutions, agents, and insurance support organizations. Increasingly, states are regulating private entities that provide utilization review (UR) for insurance companies and other payers. These regulations often include confidentiality requirements. As part of the license application process, several states require UR applicants to submit information on the organization's policies and procedures for protecting the confidentiality of individual medical records. Many states require that private UR organizations preserve the confidentiality of individual medical records and other confidential medical information obtained in the course of utilization review.

Many states require special protections for HIV status information, require informed consent for HIV testing, and make provision for anonymous testing. Some states require that counseling be made available, some require counseling prior to consent for testing, and some require that counseling be made available when test results are conveyed. Many AIDS confidentiality statutes also prohibit disclosure of HIV test results without the subject's written informed consent, subject to limited exceptions. The AIDS confidentiality statutes of most states permit AIDS-related information to be disclosed to certain medical review, infection control, or other health facility monitoring committees.

Certain federal statutes impose strict confidentiality rules on oral and written communication of records of any federally assisted program relating to drug or alcohol abuse. Authorizations to release alcohol and/or drug information must be written and must include very specific details of the consent and need for disclosure, and these written disclosures must be accompanied by a written statement prohibiting further disclosure of the released information. Such national standards may pose complications to electronic transfer of patient information for billing, UR, and other purposes.

Authorized Disclosures

In the area of generalized patient information, patients or their authorized representatives usually can authorize disclosure of confidential patient information. Generally, such consent is required for disclosure of confidential information to third-party payers. There are some exceptions to this rule, such as the consent to third-party payers for determination of payment responsibility. Facility and insurer intake registration forms should include consent to third-party reimbursement, utilization management, and quality review information access.

State law may authorize release of quality assurance (QA) or utilization information to outside review organizations, disciplinary boards, or licensing agencies. Absent such law, disclosure without consent should be avoided. The Joint Commission on Accreditation of Healthcare Organizations

(JCAHO) and other accrediting bodies require hospitals to conduct QA and UR based on review of medical records. Generally, providing such accrediting bodies access to confidential patient information without patient authorization should not create serious liability exposure.

Certain disclosures without consent are required under applicable state or local law. These may include the requirement to report child abuse, controlled substance abuse, gunshot and knife wounds and other nonaccidental injuries, unusual or suspicious deaths, births and deaths, birth defects, abortions and resulting complications, cancer, communicable diseases, and occupational diseases. The federal Unsafe Medical Devices Act requires the reporting of problems caused by unsafe medical devices.[2] Hospitals are required to report injuries from misadministration of radioactive materials, and certain other disclosures must be made to government reimbursement programs and state licensing bodies and in response to court orders and subpoenas.

Even without statutes or regulations, improper disclosure of confidential patient information could constitute invasion of privacy, breach of confidential relationship, negligence, breach of implied contract, defamation, or intentional infliction of emotional distress. Clearly, health providers and IDSs must establish protections for these documents and communications.

Securing the Information System

In establishing a secure computer information system, hospitals and MCOs should:

- Permit access only by authorized users, using passwords and key cards
- Establish and enforce policies (including sanctions) regarding disclosure or sharing of passwords, access codes, key cards, and other user identifiers
- Restrict access of each authorized user to portions of the data that are relevant to the user's functions
- Track access to records by each user to discourage unauthorized viewing
- Record and monitor attempts to gain access to the system
- Restrict use of software functions that permit certain data-copying capabilities
- Install antivirus software that can assist in detecting and blocking computer viruses and other forms of sabotage

The principal burden for protecting confidentiality of the medical relationship rests with the physician or other provider as the player closest to the physician–patient relationship. Express, written patient consent to or authorization of disclosure outside that relationship is essential. When a third party is given access, a tight description of purpose is important to control the third party's use, including protection from discovery and rediscovery to others. Those who will access confidential information should sign written confidentiality agreements, including indemnifications.

Liability Issues

Hospitals involved with the operation of an IDS may face claims for liability for alleged injuries to persons receiving health care services pursuant to an agreement between the IDS and health care purchasers, whether these purchasers are self-insured employers, third-party payers, or the government. These risks rise as hospitals take responsibility for the formation and overall operation of the IDS, and as the IDS is structurally and functionally more integrated. As a principal organizer of the IDS and a potential "deep pocket," hospitals are natural targets in such claims.

The following functions of an IDS may generate or be affected by claims of negligence:

- *Provider organization/selection:* IDS development of its panel of physicians, hospitals, and other facilities, and the provider selection criteria.
- *Financial management:* IDS management of the costs of delivering services at capitated or bundled fees or pursuant to regulated prospective fee schedules; and if the IDS becomes an HMO or other regulated MCO, the IDS' adjudication, grievance, and appeals procedures for claims.
- *Administrative services:* IDS provision of managed care contracting, human resource, purchasing, and legal and regulatory compliance services, and maintenance and repair of facilities and equipment, for its provider participants.
- *Information systems:* IDS development and implementation of information systems for systemwide data and tracking purposes.
- *Marketing:* IDS promotional services for its system and various participants.
- *Quality improvement:* IDS operation of quality review and improvement programs covering the IDS providers.
- *Utilization review:* IDS systems for ongoing UR of services provided by IDS providers to ensure appropriate intensity of service, length of stay, use of ancillary services, and so on.

Theories of Liability

Various legal theories describe the way a hospital, as an IDS member, could be liable for care delivered by others. One is *vicarious liability.* In a highly integrated system where the IDS (or parent organization or other network organization) owns or controls its service facilities and directly employs its physicians and other health care providers, the IDS may be liable for negligent acts by its physician employees and other employees providing care to patients. Although persons engaged as "independent" contractors would seem to be responsible for their own actions, many courts have found so-called independent contractor physicians to be agents of hospitals and HMOs, and likely would find them to be agents of an IDS if:

- The IDS exerts direct control over the patient's choice of physician or the physician's method of practice.
- The IDS makes "salarylike" payments to a physician.
- A patient reasonably believes that the services provided by a physician are being provided with IDS approval or under its auspices.

If physicians are deemed agents of an IDS, the IDS will be liable for the negligent acts of the physician-agent. The best way to reduce the risk of liability in a highly integrated IDS is to develop, implement, and update quality management systems and procedures.

In a less integrated IDS, the IDS should avoid establishing an employer–employee relationship, or agency relationship, with any IDS provider. Arm's-length, independent contractor relationships with providers should recognize the independence of the IDS providers. Even if the IDS must take some responsibility for providers, the risk of liability can be reduced through proper operation of quality management systems and appropriate insurance.

In its marketing materials or contracts, the IDS should avoid making representations to health plan beneficiaries that panel physicians and other providers are agents of the IDS or of any of its contract hospitals, or that the IDS takes any responsibility for the quality of care that will be provided by the *independent* physicians on the managed care panel.

If a "gatekeeper" physician is used to control specialist referrals, a referral out by the gatekeeper could raise a negligence claim if there is negligent performance by the specialist. Similarly, negligent failure to refer by a gatekeeper IDS physician can impose liability on the IDS, especially if the gatekeeper argues that IDS protocols required the nonreferral.

If the IDS operates a health plan, the plan should include mechanisms to ensure that a patient's choice of physician or other provider is not unduly limited to a closed panel. For example, the plan could include "swing-out" or point-of-service options where patients may choose a physician or other provider outside the panel at a lower reimbursement rate. Insurance regulations may limit the ability to offer these options.

Another liability theory, referred to as *corporate negligence,* holds hospitals or other institutions responsible for the negligent acts of others (physicians or other providers) because the hospital holds the provider out as competent through its medical staff credentialling and privileging process. Courts have found hospitals to be in a far better position than their patients to supervise physician performance, provide quality control, and ultimately prevent harm by withdrawing their endorsement of the provider. Similar arguments could find an IDS liable for the negligent acts of its panel of physicians and other providers.

The minimum steps a hospital or IDS should take in its physician selection and credentialing process are:

1. Investigate the qualifications of applicants, require completion of the application, and verify the accuracy of the applicant's statements, specifically with regard to his or her medical education, training, and experience.
2. Solicit information from the applicant's peers who are knowledgeable about the applicant's education, training, experience, health, competence, and ethical character.
3. Confirm current licensure and whether it currently is being challenged or is subject to limitation or restriction.
4. Review any applicant's prior involvement in an adverse malpractice action or prior loss of medical organization membership or clinical privileges at any other hospital.
5. Make a "reasonable" judgment as to approval or denial of each application after exercising ordinary care in its investigation.

The IDS should conduct appropriate provider qualification assessments and QA investigations, including peer review, for all IDS providers. Immediate and appropriate action adequate to protect patients must be the consistent discipline for any standard provider.

Whenever an IDS contracts with independent providers not subject to the IDS credentialing procedures, the contract should require adequate qualification and QA mechanisms by these providers. The IDS that designs and markets its own managed care plan must provide a sufficiently broad panel of providers from which plan beneficiaries may select physicians or other health care providers. The more limited the provider selection, the greater the IDS responsibility for panel provider competence.

Payers often try to negotiate contract terms requiring that IDSs indemnify the payer should there be negligence by any providers on the managed care panel. This is a large risk unless the IDS has adequate systems to monitor and manage service outcome quality, and has adequate insurance to bear the risk. Payers imposing their own provider qualification assessments, QA investigations, and provider selection and exclusion decisions should retain responsibility for these activities and indemnify the IDS.

Liability Arising from Cost Control Systems

Utilization review is designed to monitor quality, contain costs, and promote efficient delivery of appropriate health care services. It may be prospective, concurrent, or retrospective in nature. UR risks include defects in the

UR program design and implementation, negligence of UR personnel in administration of the UR program, and denial or delay of care to a patient.

Courts have recognized that cost controls are necessary in the health care industry, but will draw the line on cost control systems that "corrupt" sound medical judgment and compromise good patient care. Courts and juries may apportion responsibility among providers, payers, and UR organizations if each might be found to have been a "substantial factor" in a negative outcome. If UR process standards are not consistent with the community medical standards, payers and UR organizations may be liable for the harm caused.

Even if an independent UR organization conducts utilization review for the IDS, and even if the IDS is not at all involved in UR operations or decisions, the IDS might still be held liable for any harm due to the UR decisions under the theories of vicarious liability or corporate negligence (that the UR personnel were agents or under the control of the IDS).

Whether designed and operated internally or through an independent UR organization, an IDS should ensure that:

- The UR procedures meet the reasonable standards for medical decision making in the community and are updated periodically.
- The UR personnel are monitored on a continuing basis for competence and the quality of UR decisions.
- The UR program provides for assessment of all necessary information before making UR decisions.
- If possible, any independent contractor UR organization holds the IDS harmless for negligent UR decisions through an indemnity.

Generally, retrospective review by the UR has less potential for incurring liability than prospective and concurrent review.

A UR program must make timely decisions, document them adequately, and convey information effectively to any treating physician whose treatment recommendation is not endorsed by a UR team. To the greatest extent possible, the UR program should ensure that the treating physician and the patient understand that they, specifically, are responsible for making the ultimate decision regarding care, and that the UR process is only making a payment or reimbursement decision. To the extent that the IDS undertakes to provide UR and administrative claims-processing services to payers, and thus is directly involved in making coverage decisions, liability for denial or delay of care could be extended to the IDS.

Liability Arising from Managed Care Contracts

Managed care contracts held by the IDS, or managed by it and its providers, can be subject to the same claims as discussed above. However, where the

IDS, through organization and operation of a highly integrated, multiple function health care delivery system, designs and markets a "turnkey" managed health benefit plan to payers (such as self-insured employers), the IDS also risks liability based on contract, warranty, and misrepresentation. Because the IDS or its UR program is in the business of making benefit determinations, not medical decisions, most likely a personal injury claim would be handled under the federal ERISA laws.

The plan and related materials should be designed and drafted with care, particularly literature given to payers to distribute among plan enrollees and handouts about the managed care panel of providers. These plan materials may be considered to be contracts between the IDS and the payer, whose enrollees also have rights. The materials also could be interpreted to create direct contractual obligations between the IDS and the plan enrollees.

If IDS representations regarding the plan or its options imply that the IDS will provide certain types and quality of health care, failure to do so could cause legal action. This could include requiring the IDS to continue and not withhold or change the benefits. If a plan provider negligently fails to refer a patient to an appropriate specialist, or recommends an incompetent or unqualified specialist, the IDS may breach its "warranty" of delivering quality care as expressed in its marketing materials.

Another potential source of liability related to IDS plan design and operation is the payment mechanism used to compensate providers, particularly when providers receive a portion of the "savings" from reduced use of specialists or shortened hospitalization stays. In several cases, patients have argued that these financial incentives resulted in denial of needed care.

To minimize the liability arising from managed care plan contracts, the IDS could utilize qualified consultants in developing the plan's terms and conditions, particularly health care access restrictions and the financial and other incentives created. The education of marketing personnel about misrepresentations or inadvertent warranties also is important. Representations about "preferred" providers, "rigorous" credentialing and monitoring procedures, and "highest" standards of care all should be made with utmost caution. When the plan actually states that the IDS has the right to modify the plan's terms and benefits, disclaimers may be helpful.

Finally, contracts should clearly allocate the duties and responsibilities of all participants, such as who investigates the competence of the selected managed care providers and who ensures that all benefits promised under the plan are deliverable.

Under ERISA, an IDS that serves self-insured employer clients may be deemed a *fiduciary* if it provides UR, administrative claims management, or processing services, in connection with an employee health benefit plan. Therefore, all contracts should state that UR or administrative services do *not* make the IDS the plan administrator or a fiduciary as defined by ERISA. The IDS should provide claims-processing and related services only, and the employer-payer should make the final decision in all benefit and coverage disputes.

The Changing Liability Environment

The development of practice guidelines will occur at an increasing pace as IDSs undertake more risk for the quality and cost of care delivered. The development and use of guidelines, even without legislation, standardize the practice of medicine and may help establish the community norm, thus reducing the malpractice liability risk.

Future medical staff privilege applications or renewals may use new economic standards to evaluate suitability for, or renewal of, staff privileges. For example, future hospital credentials committees may examine a provider's effectiveness at utilizing medical/hospital resources. The committee would assess whether the physician has the case management skills to minimize inpatient days and has a history of avoiding care deemed unnecessary by UR criteria. An IDS may lose its contract with a regional or managed care network because it fails to apply proper economic credentialing standards to its medical providers. This trend could increase IDS exposure to liability based on delay or denial of care. Legislation has been proposed in several states to require a provider, IDS, or managed care plan to disclose its financial incentive structure and other administrative processes as part of obtaining the patient's informed consent for treatment.

Congress established the National Practitioner Data Bank to restrict the ability of incompetent physicians and dentists to move from state to state, thereby avoiding discovery of previous substandard or unprofessional conduct. The Data Bank is part of the Health Care Quality Improvement Act, whose goals also are to encourage health professional peer review and allow limited immunity for professional review activities conducted in good faith and with due process. The Data Bank is optional except to hospitals, which are required to access it during the physician credentialing process. A variety of others are permitted limited access to the Data Bank, including:

- A plaintiff's attorney in a medical malpractice suit in certain situations
- Individual licensed health care practitioners
- State licensing boards
- Federal agencies
- Utilization and quality control peer review organizations (PROs)
- HMOs and group practices conducting peer review and quality assurance programs

In the future, Data Bank information may be open to others, including patients, which could affect liability claims.

In light of liability concerns and the changing health care industry, an IDS would do well to work on creating or updating a detailed computer database and patient record and on strengthening the working relationship between its hospital and physician participants. The IDS also should plan for the rapid changes affecting governmentally funded programs and the increasingly competitive marketplace.

References

1. 42 U.S.C. § 11101.
2. 10 C.F.R. § 35.33.

Chapter 4

Contracting Issues Involving the IDS

The two basic IDS contractual arrangements are with purchasers and providers of health care services. Purchasers include employers, third-party payers, and third-party administrators (TPAs). Any third-party payer contract will include an agreement to provide a provider network and, often, certain administrative services. The IDS–payer agreement covers health services delivery and establishes a contractual reimbursement methodology. In turn, the IDS contracts with providers for these services and apportions the financial and organizational risk between itself and its providers.

IDS–Provider Contracts

Contracting issues vary according to the level of integration in the IDS among providers (hospitals, physicians, and others). Physicians often are reluctant to integrate their practice fully with other physicians, much less with a hospital. Therefore, many IDSs may simply negotiate managed care contracts on behalf of the participating providers that establish rates but do not obligate providers to act together or, sometimes, even to accept the contract. The IDS also may provide service bureau–type services to some or all of the providers, such as billing, collection, group purchasing, office management, staffing services, and so on.

If IDS providers are to meet payer requirements, they may either agree to comply with the provisions of the payer–IDS agreement (including policies and procedures on a utilization review/quality assurance [UR/QA] plan, claims payment policies, and so on) or may agree on those requirements directly with the payer. However, certain provisions, such as nondiscrimination between covered and noncovered persons and adherence to IDS policies and procedures, should be mandatory.

Some IDS–provider contracts permit the provider an "opt-in" or "opt-out" right for any payer contract executed by the IDS. Due to the uncertainty of provider acceptance of a contract, this feature clearly affects IDS ability to negotiate payer contracts and is acceptable only in a loosely integrated system and then only at an early stage. Likewise, term and termination provisions affect IDS ability to guarantee the expected provider network.

If the IDS charges the provider a network fee, the fee should relate specifically to the administrative services provided the provider by the IDS, and should be fair and reasonable. A flat fee may be preferable to one based on a percentage of billings or some other variable.

Some health care advisors disfavor exclusivity clauses because these clauses raise antitrust concerns without building loyalty. When IDSs prohibit providers from negotiating and executing contracts with third-party payers except through the IDS itself, the antitrust risks rise, particularly for loosely integrated IDS organizations. A provider-controlled IDS that is not an integrated joint venture should allow contracts with other managed care plans and health care purchasers.

The IDS should absolutely prohibit any sharing of pricing and fee information among physicians whose practices are not fully integrated. Strict confidentiality guidelines should be in place. The IDS should specifically require that individual providers not use the fee schedules of the provider network organization to influence their individual fee schedules. Competing providers must retain control over and responsibility for their own pricing decisions.

Although legal counsel can guide IDS executives through the contract review process, the following are managed care contract highlights:

- *Compensation:* How much and by whom will the IDS, the hospital, and the physicians be paid? Payment mechanisms include fee-for-service, discounted charges (by category or volume), per diem, per case or DRG (diagnosis-related group) charges, capitation (with or without risk pools), and percentage premium.
- *Mechanism of payment:* This includes timing, waiver of or variation in payment for untimely claims, appeals and penalties for late payer payment, and definition and process for paying clean claims.
- *Term:* Term and renewals with or without renegotiation of payment.
- *Termination:* Immediate, without cause, and for cause but with a time interval. Common terminations are immediate (for loss of provider license) and upon adequate notice (for loss of staff privileges, departure of the key physician(s) in a group, failure to maintain board certification, loss of Medicare provider status, loss of DEA number, termination of malpractice coverage, and so on). The IDS provider may seek to terminate immediately if the payer fails to make timely or full payment, but state law may require providers to continue care, even in the event of termination of the contract or nonpayment of the provider.
- *Parties' duties and responsibilities:* This includes direct and subcontracted services; gatekeeper roles; medical necessity determinations; specifically

restricted services in religious health systems; staff privileges in IDS facilities; manuals with binding effect; preauthorization, UR and admission/discharge protocols; insurance; and indemnifications.

- *Records:* This includes creation, maintenance, destruction, confidentiality, and proprietary value; access, copying, and storage.
- *Assignment:* Is an assignment of the contract without consent of the other party permitted?
- *Insolvency issues:* Are there protections in place in the event that a party experiences financial problems?
- *Third-party beneficiary:* Does the hospital have any rights as to contracts between another provider and the IDS? Does the payer?
- *Publicity:* Who can publicize membership in the IDS, and how?
- *Regulatory reform:* Should state or regulatory reform make portions of the contract ill-advised or even illegal, how is legal review performed, and should arbitration be required before termination?

IDS–Payer Contracts

Typically, an IDS packages the services of the providers into a product that the payer wishes to buy. For hospitals and other providers, it may be "seller beware." The IDS should carefully analyze the payer's enrollee base, payment and financial history, license status, reputation, and method of doing business. Due diligence is essential to verify payer representations, and periodic checks should be maintained.

An IDS–payer contract under consideration may assume that the IDS's individual providers are contractually required to perform certain services or adhere to certain conditions, when in fact they are not. To facilitate payer contract negotiations, an IDS needs the most flexibility possible in its individual provider agreements. To the extent possible, payer and provider contracts should contain common language, terms, and obligations. This allows passing provider commitments to payers and passing payer commitments down to providers without lengthy legal counsel review.

Compensation concerns include licensure questions if capitation, prepayment, or other financial arrangements shift risk from payer to IDS, and other issues reviewed earlier in chapter 2.

If the IDS cannot obtain an annual or periodic opportunity to renegotiate rates, it should seek favorable term lengths and not-for-cause termination rights. The IDS should negotiate for financial incentives for prompt payment and increases in patient volume, control of coordination of benefits situations, and the right to seek reimbursement from other possible payment sources. In the unfortunate event of payer bankruptcy, the providers and the IDS need access to any available payment source. (The patients likely will be protected by a "hold harmless" clause in their participation agreement.)

The role of both IDS and payer in provider credentialling must be clear. The payer may want the right to veto or terminate a specific provider. The payer also may want a guarantee of the quality, qualifications, and continued availability of the providers on the panel. As these requirements become common, they must be coordinated carefully with any provider rights to procedural due process described in the provider agreement. In addition, the IDS must be very careful not to promise a specific provider panel if providers are permitted (under their own individual contracts) to opt out of a payer contract or to terminate their participation at will. The IDS and providers could agree that the IDS would identify subpanels of providers in accordance with precise criteria.

Important payer responsibilities include:

- Providing the terms of its benefit plans to the IDS organization, along with a right of termination in case of material changes
- Providing financial incentives for its covered persons or beneficiaries to use network providers (for example, greater coverage and reduced copayments and deductibles)
- Identifying beneficiaries and verifying eligibility and coverage
- Paying claims in a timely manner, with penalties, termination, and utilization review and dispute resolution detailed
- Obtaining patient consents for release of medical records to the payer and the IDS, with provider rights to verification

Essential definitions in the IDS–payer contract include:

- Covered services, including any applicable deductibles or copayments and a mechanism to notify the IDS of any changes prior to the effective date.
- Medical necessity, including the review process and appeal process for both physician and patient, and indemnification from the payer should the physician alter the patient's treatment plan based on payer requirements.
- Emergency services.
- Limitations for preexisting conditions and/or experimental procedures, including the scope and the standard to be applied.
- Multiple plans, including clear explanations of each of the variations, perhaps in attachments to the contract, and a requirement for written notification of any changes.
- Standards of care.
- UR/QA procedures, including the mechanism for appeals and prior adequate written notice.
- Insurance and indemnification, avoiding unintended or overly broad obligations. (Generally, the contractual assumption of risk or indemnification of another party is outside standard insurance policy coverage, so written confirmation from the carrier is necessary.)

- Public relations: The payer will want to be able to identify the IDS and/or its providers in promotional literature. The IDS should try to retain the right to approve (or at least review) these materials prior to their release. Alternatively, the contract should specify by category the types of materials that will identify the IDS. If the IDS wants to publicize its affiliation with a payer, the contract should convey this right. The consent process concerning marketing should be clear in the contract.
- Compliance with applicable governmental and professional standards: The payer should provide assurances that it will maintain in good standing all licenses, accreditations, certifications, or approvals necessary to operate and that it will conduct its business in a manner consistent with all applicable governmental and professional standards. It will seek a reciprocal provision from the IDS.
- Term and termination: If the initial term is more than one year, a requirement might be considered to review the rates annually. Termination without cause usually requires a lengthy notice period (up to six months), whereas termination with cause can occur on an accelerated basis, such as 30 days with notice. *Cause* should be defined in the contract.
- Future legal developments: Depending on state law, the uncertain effects of future events could be addressed through termination provisions, elimination of some contract clauses (keeping the remainder), and/or a provision that requires the parties to use best efforts to enter negotiations promptly to modify the agreement.
- Dispute resolution: The contract should describe procedures for three general types of potential disputes: patient grievances, usually concerning coverage; provider grievances, which can be about payment issues or credentialing; and disputes between organization and payer about contract terms.

Administrative Services Agreements: Selected Issues

The IDS may provide administrative services to the payer under an ASO (administrative service organization) agreement or be referred to as a TPA (third-party administrator) or both. TPA services could include UR, QA, claims processing, and related services. Increasingly, IDSs are finding that expertise in such areas enhances patient flow and management. IDS expertise may start with managing its own employee benefit plan.

The major issues related to ASO arrangements include:

- *Consistency with other agreements:* The ASO agreement needs to be consistent with any separate IDS–payer agreement and the applicable provider agreements.
- *Contracting party:* When providing TPA services, the IDS should contract with the employer or plan sponsor, not with the payer; or the IDS

should be recognized in the payer contract with the employer/plan sponsor contractor as the provider of TPA services.

- *Payment from general assets:* Payments to the IDS for TPA services should be made from the general assets of the employer/sponsor, not from the plan assets.
- *Denial of plan fiduciary status:* The ASO agreement should state specifically that the IDS-TPA is not the plan administrator or a fiduciary as defined by ERISA. The payer should make the final decision in all benefit and coverage disputes.
- *Payment of claims:* The most common claims payment methods are:
  - A payer-funded "escrow account" from which the TPA draws down amounts to pay claims
  - Periodic money transfers by the payer to the TPA to make payments to providers or covered persons
  - Direct payments by the payer to providers or covered persons on advice from the TPA
- *Compliance with state insurance, licensure, and other laws:* These were discussed in chapter 2.
- *Protection against benefit denial claims:* The payer should agree that it will defend, indemnify, and hold the IDS-TPA harmless, and the IDS should obtain adequate errors and omissions (E&O) insurance, with the IDS-TPA and its providers named as additional insureds on the payer's E&O insurance policy.
- *Access and ownership of records between TPA and plan:* These issues can involve privacy, malpractice liability, access to information affecting bidding of the payer contract, and, ultimately, the ease with which the payer can terminate the ASO agreement and contract with another IDS.

Special Medicaid Managed Care Contracting Issues

The market transition from traditional Medicaid fee for service to Medicaid managed care translates into three significant types of opportunities for private and public health care organizations: development of additional private Medicaid HMOs; development of Medicaid capability among commercial HMOs; and development of public Medicaid HMOs. Specialized waivers are required for Medicaid managed care contracting. State Medicaid programs are implementing managed care approaches to improve access to needed care while controlling costs. The Arizona plan, the Oregon plan, TennCare, and the California initiative have led state reform initiatives. Congressional reforms of the Medicaid program are likely to have a significant effect on these developments.

If a state is operating under a managed care waiver, HMOs that are federally qualified or that meet state plan HMO criteria may contract to provide comprehensive services to Medicaid beneficiaries on a prepaid basis, when preapproved by the Health Care Financing Administration (HCFA). Comprehensive services are one of the following:

- Inpatient hospital services, plus at least one of the following:
  - Physician services
  - Outpatient hospital services
  - Skilled nursing facility services
  - EPSDT (early pregnancy screening, detection, and treatment) services
  - Home health services
  - Laboratory and X-ray services
  - Rural or community health clinic services
- Three or more of the services listed above

Prepaid health plans (PHPs) are entities that provide services to Medicaid recipients on a prepaid basis but do not contract to provide "comprehensive services." An example is a hospital that contracts to provide specific services such as neonatal care or preventive care networks. Requirements for PHPs do not include state HMO plan requirements and, in general, are more flexible than those for HMOs. In some states, there are no PHPs other than licensed HMOs. One possible reason is that in the absence of a comprehensive program, both the state and providers have been reluctant to enter into risk-bearing contracts that may improve services but, due to selection issues, may also substantially increase the overall costs and, therefore, the financial risk of providing these services.

Primary care case management programs (PCCMs) typically involve medical groups or clinics that contract on a prepaid basis to provide less than comprehensive services to Medicaid beneficiaries. In such programs, the state generally contracts directly with non-PCCM providers such as hospitals and retains at a minimum the utilization risk for those services. States may establish PCCMs under which Medicaid recipients are assigned to a primary care physician who serves as a *gatekeeper,* that is, the primary care physician authorizes all care received by recipients assigned to him or her. A freedom of choice waiver under Section 1915(b) of the Social Security Act is required to permit assignment of recipients to primary care physicians under a PCCM.

Individual providers or networks of providers may participate in Medicaid managed care by contracting with HMOs, PHPs, or PCCMs as a part of a provider network. Contracts may be on a fee-for-service basis, or the plans may subcapitate providers, meaning that the provider accepts an actuarially determined portion of the plan's capitated payment as payment in full for its services. Because these contracts are not directly with the state, the individual provider is free from state fee schedules and restrictions in negotiating its reimbursement from the Medicaid managed care entities. Sometimes providers must accept their reimbursement as payment in full without recourse if the entity fails financially (state law may so require). In most contracts, the provider is required to preauthorize hospitalizations and certain outpatient procedures. Some states require IDS organizations that accept capitation and include multiple types of providers, such as hospitals and physicians, to obtain an HMO license. Some states provide "model subcontracts" that will not trigger the HMO licensure requirement.

Many states permit providers to accept prepayment directly from the Medicaid program for their services, if for less than "comprehensive services." Generally, such contracts are restricted to hospitals or physician groups providing a limited range of services.

By law, Medicaid recipients must be free to obtain medical services from any provider qualified to perform that service, absent a federal waiver of the requirement. However, the state can "lock in" a recipient for the first six months of his or her enrollment and restrict "at will" disenrollment from certain HMOs.

At least 25 percent of all enrollees of Medicaid-participating HMOs must be individuals who are not eligible for Medicare or Medicaid. A number of exceptions to this requirement are available, most notably for public HMOs and for the first three years of operation of a new HMO. Individual waivers for particular HMOs also have been obtained from the U.S. Department of Health and Human Services (DHHS).

The cost of Medicaid risk contracts may not exceed the cost to Medicaid of providing the same services, on a fee-for-service basis, to an actuarially equivalent population. States have considerable discretion to determine equivalent costs under this formula. It is likely that these historical costs do not include the cost of preventive services that the HMO is required to offer. Once states have a capitation program in operation in a given area for a period of time, fee-for-service data available for comparative purposes in order to establish the upper-payment limit will inevitably decrease. This may lead to comparisons with noncomparable populations, costs, and services.

In general, Medicaid recipients enrolled in a comprehensive managed care program may disenroll voluntarily without cause at any time. Even where a freedom of choice waiver is obtained, recipients must have at least one option to disenroll from an HMO to another plan, such as another HMO, a PHP, a PCCM, or fee-for-service coverage.

The Medicaid fraud laws limit the financial incentive arrangements that HMOs may enter into with participating physicians. Managed care programs also are subject to civil monetary penalties if they fail to substantially furnish medically necessary services covered under the state Medicaid plan.

Capitated rates may be subject to change with little or no notice based on factors over which the plan has no control, such as state budget shortfalls or reductions in federal matching funds. Additionally, capitated rates may not reflect increases in fee-for-service rates until years after the increases go into effect. Stop-loss protection, if available at affordable rates, should be considered not only for high-cost hospitalizations, but also on a disease-specific basis, such as for patients with AIDS.

Because Medicaid recipients may enroll and disenroll voluntarily without cause, and because frequent changes in eligibility lead to involuntary disenrollment, a turnover rate as high as 40 percent a year could be experienced, particularly in the early years of participation before a plan is well established. Unless clearly provided otherwise in the Medicaid contract, a managed care plan could find itself at risk for retroactive eligibility determinations, even if those determinations are the result of errors made by the Medicaid program.

To participate effectively in a Medicaid managed care contract, a plan or provider network must have sufficient providers who are willing to treat Medicaid patients and who are located in areas accessible to the Medicaid population. For plans that have previously contracted with commercial payers only, this may mean recruiting new providers in new geographic areas and finding physicians or other providers to provide a substantial amount of care to Medicaid enrollees. Hospital coverage is unlimited, transportation is required, and dental benefits often are covered, adding to the provider contracting burden.

Medicaid recipients moving to a managed care plan from a fee-for-service system are likely to be unfamiliar with the principles of preventive care and unaccustomed to seeking treatment from primary care physicians. The hospital emergency room is a common source of care for many inner-city Medicaid recipients. A considerable investment of resources in patient services may be required to change traditional patterns of utilization, increase levels of preventive care, and reduce the incidence of out-of-plan care. Moreover, patient services related to health prevention and health education, well-baby care, and so on may be required at a much greater level than is generally required for a commercial population.

Additional Books of Interest

➤ A time-saving overview of 15 current management methods.

Today's Management Methods: A Guide for the Health Care Executive
Robert G. Gift, MS, and Catherine F. Kinney, PhD, Editors

This easy-to-read reference from the AHA is exactly what the busy health care executive needs. It gives you concise, in-depth discussions of 15 effective management methods being used today, and it helps you evaluate each within the framework of your organization. Whether you're trying to get a broad picture of current management methods or simply need a quick encapsulation of a particular method, this book is for you.

Catalog No. E99-001117 (must be included when ordering)
1996. 324 pages, 60 figures, 14 tables.
$69.00 (AHA members, $55.00)

➤ An executive tool for building a solid information technology program.

The CEO's Guide to Health Care Information Systems
by Joseph M. DeLuca, FACHE, with Rebecca Enmark Cagan of JDA

This reference book provides the busy executive with an understanding of the current state of information systems (IS) and information technology (IT) and how it can support emerging needs in the health care marketplace. This book briefs you on what you need to know to become more effective in your leadership role. And when questions arise, you'll know where to turn for more information.

Catalog No. E99-093105 (must be included when ordering)
1996. 128 pages, 14 figures, 15 tables.
$40.00 (AHA members, $32.00)